Health issues and adol

Most research and policy agendas relating to young people are dominated by adult concerns about young people's health; rarely are the issues looked at from young people's perspectives. Numerous public health campaigns target young people's drinking, smoking, drug-taking and sexual behaviour, despite the fact that this is the segment of the population with the lowest morbidity and mortality of any age. Do young people themselves share this concern about their health? This gap in our knowledge may be a critical factor in explaining some of the problems that health educators face in getting young people to transform health knowledge into action.

With their own research as a base, Shucksmith and Hendry set adult agendas to one side and explore young people's own views about their health and health behaviours. They provide recommendations about initiatives relevant to a wide range of professionals and researchers involved in the health education of young people. *Health Issues and Adolescents* will be invaluable for health educators, policy makers and all professionals interested in developing strategies which include young people as real participants in decision-making.

Janet Shucksmith is Senior Lecturer in Sociology, University of Aberdeen. **Leo Hendry** is Professor of Education, University of Aberdeen and Professor of Psychology, Norwegian University of Science and Technology, Trondheim. Their previous publications include *Young People's Leisure and Lifestyles* (1993).

Adolescence and Society
Series editor: John C. Coleman
The Trust for the Study of Adolescence

The general aim of the series is to make accessible to a wide readership the growing evidence relating to adolescent development. Much of this material is published in relatively inaccessible professional journals, and the goals of the books in this series will be to summarize, review and place in context current work in the field so as to interest and engage both an undergraduate and a professional audience.

The intention of the authors is to raise the profile of adolescent studies among professionals and in institutions of higher education. By publishing relatively short, readable books on interesting topics to do with youth and society, the series will make people more aware of the relevance of the subject of adolescence to a wide range of social concerns.

The books will not put forward any one theoretical viewpoint. The authors will outline the most prominent theories in the field and will include a balanced and critical assessment of each of these. Whilst some of the books may have a clinical or applied slant, the majority will concentrate on normal development.

The readership will rest primarily in two major areas: the undergraduate market, particularly in the fields of psychology, sociology and education; and the professional training market, with particular emphasis on social work, clinical and educational psychology, counselling, youth work, nursing and teacher training.

Also available in this series

Adolescent Health
Patrick C. L. Heaven

Identity in Adolescence
Jane Kroger

The Nature of Adolescence (second edition)
John C. Coleman and Leo Hendry

The Adolescent in the Family
Patricia Noller and Victor Callan

Young People's Understanding of Society
Adrian Furnham and Barrie Stacey

Growing up with Unemployment
Anthony H. Winefield, Marika Tiggermann, Helen R. Winefield and Robert D. Goldney

Young People's Leisure and Lifestyles
Leo B. Hendry, Janet Shucksmith, John G. Love and Anthony Glendinning

Sexuality in Adolescence
Susan Moore and Doreen Rosenthal

Adolescent Gambling
Mark Griffiths

Adolescent Health
Patrick C. L. Heaven

Youth, AIDS, and Sexually Transmitted Diseases
Susan Moore, Doreen Rosenthal and Anne Mitchell

Fathers and Adolescents
Shmuel Shulman and Inge Seiffge-Krenke

Health issues and adolescents

adolescents

Growing up, speaking out

Janet Shucksmith and Leo B. Hendry

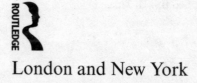

London and New York

First published 1998
by Routledge
11 New Fetter Lane, London EC4P 4EE

Simultaneously published in the USA and Canada by Routledge
29 West 35th Street, New York, NY 10001

Typeset in Times by RefineCatch Limited, Bungay, Suffolk
Printed and bound in Great Britain by Clays Ltd, St. Ives PLC

British Library Cataloguing in Publication Data
A catalogue record for this book is available from the British Library

Library of Congress Cataloging in Publication Data
Shucksmith, Janet
    Health issues and adolescents: growing up, speaking out / Janet
Shucksmith and Leo B.Hendry.
        p.   cm. – (Adolescence and society)
    Includes bibliographical references and index.
    1. Teenagers – Health and hygiene.   2. Health attitudes.
  3. Teenagers – Attitudes.   4. Health behavior in adolescence.
  5. Teenagers – Health and hygiene – Scotland.   6. Health attitudes –
  Scotland.   7. Teenagers – Scotland – Attitudes.   8. Health behavior
  in adolescence – Scotland.   I. Hendry, Leo B.   II. Title.
  III. Series.
  RJ47.53.S455   1998
  613′.0433 – dc21   97–46525

ISBN 0–415–16848–1 (hbk)
ISBN 0–415–16849–X (pbk)

Contents

Foreword

This book represents an important and novel approach to studying young people's own self-defined health issues. Despite the acknowledged relevance for health promotion and policy of listening to lay views and understanding the salience of health concerns in people's daily lives, less attention has been paid to the views and agendas of young people themselves. I was, therefore, very pleased when several of my then colleagues in the Programmes Division at the Health Education Board for Scotland acknowledged this research need and agreed jointly to fund a strategic qualitative study.

The research team from the Centre for Educational Research, University of Aberdeen, was enthusiastic and inventive in their methods of researching with young people and carried out the study in a refreshingly open and flexible manner. It was a pleasure to work with them and with the other members of the advisory committee. Carrying out good qualitative research involves working with research participants in a sensitive and mutually respectful manner so that meaningful data can be constructed. I consider that this study had those qualities; and that this is reflected in the vividness of the accounts from young people of their lives, which are represented in this book.

Although research *about* health-relevant behaviours in youth has proliferated during the past decade, such work has usually explored 'adultist' ideas about health concerns and employed predominantly quantitative methods. Often these health-relevant behaviours have also been documented separately from an understanding of their meaning and salience in young people's lives as a whole. In addition, there has been a tendency to present young people as a homogeneous group, with little feel for the variety of their views and experiences. The study reported in this book, therefore, provides a refreshingly different qualitative perspective on young people's health concerns; one which is grounded in an appreciation of the varied lives which they experience in Scotland in the 1990s.

Dr Kathryn Backett-Milburn
Research Unit of Health and Behavioural Change, University of Edinburgh (formerly at Health Education Board for Scotland)

Acknowledgements

In completing this book we are grateful for the support and collaboration of a number of people and organisations, and would wish to record our thanks to them here. First, thanks go to the Health Education Board for Scotland for providing us with a research grant to carry out the work reported here, and for the encouragement and support of their officers throughout the study. Second, we must thank Dr Kathryn Backett-Milburn and the members of our advisory committee for their advice and erudition. We also give thanks to Ann Brodie, Margaret Sinclair and Nikki Strachan for the range of secretarial help supplied through the course of this work.

We are especially grateful to Sheila Wood and to Guy Dewsbury, who were the field officers on the project. Without their organisation and excellent manner in the field we would have been unable to access young people's voices as well. Thanks are also due to the schools across Scotland who co-operated with us on this work. They are unnamed in order to protect the confidentiality of the final group that we must acknowledge. To all the young people who 'spoke out' and provided us with such valuable views on their lives, experiences, health concerns and relationships – thank you.

1 Young people's perceptions of their own health needs

Introduction

Young people, in the main, are notoriously and ridiculously healthy. For many years the low mortality and morbidity in this age group meant that it was largely ignored by epidemiologists and health scientists in favour of those groups in early childhood or middle to later life where there were enough sick or dying people to make it worth counting and watching patterns.

What has become clearer in recent years, however, as a consequence of the intrusion of the notion of healthy lifestyle into such debates and the changing emphasis to prevention of ill-health, is that many of the health behaviours evident in young people, while not having serious consequences at that stage, may be the precursors of patterns of illness or affliction in later years. If we want to tackle the rates of heart disease or the level of bronchial problems in the middle-aged or elderly we may have to start our preventive work with the habits and beliefs of the young. For example, several studies suggest that physical activity 'tracks' across adolescence into adulthood (Dishman and Dunn, 1989; Anderssen *et al.*, 1994).

What is also clear from the more sophisticated disaggregation of global statistics is that many of the patterns of behaviour which are inherently problematic are clustered within certain groups in the population or are associated with one another through complex routes of choice and decision-making as well as by the variation in the way in which structural factors such as class, race and gender impinge on populations.

Understanding of the importance of young people's health is now formally enshrined in the performance targets set in documents such as *The Health of the Nation* (Secretary of State for Health, 1991). How are health educators and other professionals with a responsibility for young people's health and welfare to attack these challenges? It was felt by several of the agencies responsible for health education that a crucial element in the formulation of strategy was an understanding of how young people themselves viewed health and health-related issues. Moreover, it was seen to be important to collect data on this topic not through the sort of quantitative survey that delivers aggregate statistics on behaviours like smoking, but through a qualitative study which would allow young people the opportunity to comment on health issues as they were experienced by them on a day-to-day level. Data of this sort might help health educators to formulate interventions or programmes for young people which were salient, realistic and better targeted.

Young people's perceptions of their own health needs

This book sets out to report the findings from a project commissioned by the Health Education Board for Scotland in 1994 in order to provide empirical findings concerning young people's perceptions of their own health needs. The research aims were, broadly, to allow adolescents aged 15 years to identify and discuss their own health needs within the context of their daily lives over a period of time, and thus to provide in-depth information, both generic and specific, which would assist the development of effective and culturally appropriate health promotion initiatives with adolescents.

From this a set of specific research objectives were derived. Amongst them were the following:

- to explore adolescent health issues and health promotion needs without a pre-defined adult agenda;
- to understand the place of behaviours which may have health implications within the context of adolescent lifestyles;
- further to investigate linkages between youth culture and health-relevant behaviours.

• critically to assess the role of 'adultist' definitions in the shaping of adolescent health problems; and to reflect on how this process impacts on the effectiveness of health promotion.

Putting young people at the centre

The major intention behind the project was, then, to allow young people in mid-adolescence to 'speak for themselves' about health issues and concerns without a pre-defined adult agenda. How unusual a remit was this?

'Children are all foreigners. We treat them as such', R. W. Emerson (1803–1882) is quoted as saying. This quote is used by Jane Ribbens (1995) to point to the extent to which analyses of childhood have often sought to define children in relation to the more familiar world of adulthood. Children are typically construed as 'Other' than adult (Ribbens, 1995: 61), and it is only recently perhaps that children and their needs and perceptions have begun to be seriously and systematically studied in their own right. Recent work has begun to turn away from the old conceptualisation of children as merely 'adults in training', which inevitably focused interest on the socialisation processes of childhood and adolescence. Researchers and policy-makers have, too, ceased to focus on the extreme, the perverse, the exotic, and have started, in Qvortrup's (1995) opinion, to become interested in the typical, normal and common conditions for the majority of children.

Why this should be so is a matter of conjecture. Qvortrup (1995) toys with the idea that the catalyst for such a shift in the paradigm is the public perception that childhood itself has become something of a social problem or has started to be seen as a source of social problems. The actual behaviour of children and young people may have changed less than our interpretation of those behaviours.

Perhaps the positive outcome of this concern will be a change in what Kaufmann (1990) has called a structural disregard or structural indifference *vis-à-vis* children and their families. Qvortrup (1995) comments on the fact that children do not have any defenders or lobbyists, or, comparatively speaking, very weak ones. It is hard to hear their own voices above the babble of those who speak on their behalf or interpret their experience for them. Mayall makes a similar point:

> Children do not on the whole speak for themselves. They are spoken for, by adults. And it is adults who have constructed the understandings about what children are which serve as the bases for the lives children lead.   (1994: 2)

Mayall's statement precedes a discussion in which she demonstrates how Western European policies and practices towards children treat them as essentially pre-social beings who are somehow 'less' than adults in terms of skills, competence and knowledge, and who must, as a consequence, be regarded as vulnerable, innocent and in need of adult protection. In an interesting discussion she traces how our policies have always reflected the academic traditions of psychology (which stress developmentalism) and sociology (which stress socialisation), rather than, say, anthropology, which looks across cultures and throws up challenging models across time and across geographical space of societies where children were and are viewed quite differently (James and Prout, 1990; Joseph, 1993).

Our protective behaviour towards our children, stemming from this model, is benevolent, of course, but a necessary concomitant is that we have reserved for ourselves the right to make decisions on their behalf, thus robbing them of the chance to have a say in many of the major decisions which affect their lives. This is as true in the realm of health education as in any other sphere of our social lives.

Kalnins *et al.* (1992) suggest that we need to create a shift in our thinking about children as recipients of health promotion to thinking of children as partners, whose views are valid in their own right. Part of the problem in performing this shift is clearly the difficulty most adults have in 'accepting children's competence' (Kalnins *et al.*, 1992: 58). Some might see this situation as having many similarities to the great shift in thinking that has taken place over the roles either of women or of various ethnic groups in society (Qvortrup, 1990). In the first case the protective paternalism that was designed to shield women from any worry, trouble and aggravation that they might have struggled to cope with has many resonances in the language which we use to explain our rationale for doing the agenda-setting on health (and in other areas) on behalf of our children. Lewis and Lewis (1982), commenting on the dearth of research in America up until about ten years ago on this topic, note that social values and norms also may be reflected in what is *not* studied. They feel that, although science may not be blind, individuals and scientists often fail to recognise or think about the unfamiliar.

In recent years this 'child blindness' has been eroded somewhat by a variety of factors. Levin (1989), for instance, in discussing the need to involve young people not just in the process of consultation, but also the process of decision-making about health, states that it is essential, therefore, that policy formulation be fundamentally a public process with continuous inputs from young people as well as from those who claim to represent them.

Such ideas have been advocated strongly in relation to the relatively new field of health education for young people on the topic of HIV/AIDS. Aggleton *et al.* (1992), for instance, comment on the need for participatory needs assessment as a prerequisite for future work with young people. Focus group work involving young people directly in the agenda-setting process and leading to the identification of intervention priorities, they feel, should precede any local HIV/AIDS health promotion initiative. They state clearly that, while the views of teachers, parents, youth leaders and other adults may be sought, they should never be afforded priority over the express needs of young people themselves. We might doubt whether such an ideal would work in practice. Young people would have a very different (and possibly unacceptable) agenda from Aggleton and even from themselves ten years on, but the point about the need for consultation is, nevertheless, a valid one.

This issue has been brought to a finer focus recently by the attempt of a number of different agencies and authors to review progress on the implementation in the European context of the United Nations Convention on the Rights of the Child. An example is the draft Scottish Agenda for children (CRDU, 1994). Taking as one of its main themes 'Health and Health Care services', the Agenda attempts to translate the general recommendations of the United Nations Convention on the Rights of the Child (to which Britain is a signatory) into a Scottish policy context. In examining children's rights within the health context, the Agenda draws attention to Article 12 of the UN Convention which makes it clear that children and young people have the right to express their views, and to have those views taken into account. This relates not only to matters concerning their individual medical treatment, but also to 'the rights of children and young people, as a consumer group in the community, to participate in the planning of health services' (chapter 3, p. 1).

The work of Jones and Wallace (1992), at a theoretical level, has again emphasised young people's need to have better rights as citizens if they are to develop as responsible members of the community. They state:

> The imposition of dependency status on many young people who in other historical or social circumstances might be able to live independent lives, takes away adult responsibility and places young people under the legal control of their parents. Their rights to freedom and self-determination are thus restricted. So too are their responsibilities. Thus, at a time when both independence and responsibilities should be increasing, they are not. Yet rights and responsibilities are inextricably linked . . . .   (1992: 154)

Some commentators have been wary of these developments. Waiton (1995), for instance, argues that it is essentially a paternalistic strategy to offer to define and frame rights *on behalf of,* rather than *with,* young people. That the children's rights movement fails to engage with youth cultures is clear (Hendry *et al.*, 1995), and it may, in fact, be dissonant with currents such as the 'right to party' and the 'hedonism for hard times' suggested by Redhead and other commentators on rave culture (Redhead, 1993). Little of the pressure to participate is coming from young people themselves. We do not live now in an age of student protest or popular outcry from young people. For the most part young people are disenfranchised by poverty or by institutional structures and have no coherent voice or lobby.

Moreover there are some authors who are wary of the whole 'rights and relevance' movement with regard to children, not because they resist the idea that children are competent to express preferences or to take part in decision-making, but because they see the focus on 'youth' as a distraction from an understanding of the heterogeneity of the mass of young people. Frost and Stein (1992), for example, argue that young people experience powerlessness through their status as young people by exclusion from decision-making processes in schools, or, on a wider basis, by their exclusion from the political process. However they feel that this powerlessness is overlaid by other categories, most notably social class, disability, ethnicity and gender which interact with generation to produce a matrix of power and powerlessness.

Chisholm and du Bois Raymond (1993) in studying youth in a European context similarly argue that the transitions from youth to adulthood are complex, fragmented and heavily influenced by systematic social inequalities. It behoves us to remember this as we move through the empirical data presented here. Although we will inevitably generalise about young people's experiences and beliefs we must also accept the variety of experience and understanding that young people will exhibit.

Some of the rationale for this new interest in listening to young people's views must lie in the recognition that existing health education messages and interventions are increasingly shown to have little impact on the actual behaviour of large segments of the youth population. Smoking rates amongst young people demonstrate a hard core of smokers resistant to every form of media campaign, for example. Information campaigns about HIV are shown to raise knowledge levels, yet risky sexual behaviours are still commonplace. Drug culture seems to embed itself more firmly among youth whether health promoters advocate 'say no' strategies or seek a harm-minimisation approach.

As information approaches have been shown to fail in terms of transforming behaviour, health promotion has turned more and more to methods which seek to develop skills or to impart strategies that can be used by young people. The emphasis of much such work is on individuals accepting personal responsibility for their health and having both the knowledge and skills to make decisions appropriately. The focus on empowerment and autonomy in health promotion is strangely at odds with many other currents in British society. For, despite overt attempts to convince us that young people's interests are paramount (as in the passing of the Children Act 1989) young people are not seen within the welfare system as having the potential to exercise considered judgement or autonomy. Thus 16-year-old people in the UK, whatever their circumstances, have no entitlement to social security support. It is envisaged that forcing families to assume responsibility for young people into their twenties will both transform 'family values' and relieve the state of the responsibility for social policy in relation to the young (Hendry *et al.*, 1995).

Brannen *et al.* (1994) also found occasion in their work to dredge up the hoary old problem of social control of young people. Davis (1990) and others have documented the extent to which youth is asked to 'carry the can' when all is not well with the economic or moral well-being of the nation. We live in such times currently, and parents are continually being exhorted to take more responsibility for the actions and attitudes of their offspring. This is difficult for both parents and teenage offspring to negotiate when there are also these countervailing forces suggesting that young people should be empowered and made autonomous:

> The current emphasis upon parental responsibility in controlling young people's anti-social behaviour occurs in an economic climate in which young people's future, in terms of job opportunities, is bleak. It is also a moral climate in which the rights and responsibilities of community and citizenship have been ousted in favour of the values of the marketplace. Parents are being required to fill an economic and a moral vacuum. Yet they appear to have little or no role within a model of health education which emphasises the individual responsibility of young people for their own actions.
>
> (Brannen *et al.*, 1994: 214)

Perhaps the greatest challenge to the notion of putting children at the heart of things comes from those people, many of them parents, who have only their young people's welfare at heart. Qvortrup notes:

> Claims for the extension of rights to new groups have always involved a challenge to 'common sense', to the 'ordinary man'

or to the 'natural' social order. Generally long periods pass by from the launching of a cause to the implementation of its aims . . . . To raise questions of oppression seems, however, to be a necessary pre-condition for solving the problem, even if for the time being it may appear politically naive.

(1990: 78)

Within the reports of the work which follow, an attempt is made to allow young people's voices to come through strongly.

The structure of the book

The next chapter looks *generally* at the methods or ways in which we can explore young people's own agendas on health and *specifically* at the methods used to gather data in this study. Beyond this, the chapters present the empirical data from the project. In presenting the data it was the authors' clear intention to avoid the topic-by-topic presentation of findings (smoking, sexual health, drug misuse and so on) that characterises so many books about health or health education. To have done so would have been to ignore the sense of what came through from young people's accounts. A systematic way – but one which did not destroy the integrity of the accounts – seemed to be one which looked at the different levels of influence that impinged on young people's understanding of health. Thus we have tried to move from the level of broad cultural influences on young people and their understanding of health, through the level of local neighbourhood influences and peer group norms on health beliefs, to the micro level of family interaction and transmission of belief.

In some instances we have tried to manage the vast volume of data that a qualitative study generates by focusing on one particular issue that can be used to characterise the way in which influence at that level operates. Thus in chapter 2 we start by focusing on the influence of broad social cultures on issues around dieting and body image. Throughout the text we have referred to other studies where these provide a context or background for the results presented here, or where the results from other work seem to confirm or challenge our own findings. This level of interpretation seems to us entirely necessary if the results are to be seen to have wider validity and to be of use to policy-makers, but we hope that in doing so we have not lost the immediacy of young people's own accounts.

The book concludes with a chapter on the implications of the study for all those with a professional or academic interest in the health and welfare of young people.

2 'Giving a voice to children'
Exploring young people's own agendas on health

Introduction

In this chapter we examine the ways in which we can set about exploring young people's own views about health and giving them a voice of their own on health issues. In the first section we review how difficult it is to trace young people's own concerns in much of the writing about adolescent health, and we look at the advantages and disadvantages of different research methods for allowing young people's own concerns to be heard. We follow this with an account of the research design and methods used in the study described in this book.

Problems in exploring young people's own agendas about health

Survey data

Much of the current information on health habits such as smoking and drinking and on health attitudes and perceptions has been gathered by means of large-scale representative surveys using self-completion questionnaires. This raises questions about the validity or truthfulness of some of the information volunteered by young people. Individuals may have reasons either for exaggerating behaviours which (to them) seem admirable, or for concealing behaviours, attitudes or prejudices which may be illegal or strongly condemned by society generally or the peer group in particular. Belief in the confidentiality of such research methods is often far from absolute. Additionally, these surveys are usually planned and implemented from an adultist – rather than from a young person's – perspective.

Further caveats have to be issued with regard to the comparability of surveys. The form of question will clearly influence the type of response given and too little attention is paid to this fact in the reporting of many surveys. Then, too, it is difficult to interpret the definitional boundaries or categories in some studies. 'Heavy smokers', for example, may be differently defined in studies, making comparability difficult.

Such survey data serve a purpose in keying us into general trends, but it is really in the *disaggregation* of the figures that facts of real importance emerge. Which is more interesting as a fact – that 18 per cent of all 15-year-olds smoke, or that significantly more girls than boys smoke at this age; that smoking peaks at this age and thereafter declines, or that youngsters in certain socioeconomic groups are more likely to smoke? Certainly, in targeting health promotion or evaluating where field interventions might be focused it is the disaggregated figures that are more illuminating. Methodological problems raise their head, however, in attempting to pursue this to its logical conclusion. Even large-scale nationally representative surveys have difficulty in producing results down to the local level (for instance, of a school catchment or neighbourhood) and in illustrating differences which are statistically significant, simply because of the small cell sizes at these levels. Some health behaviours and beliefs, notably those related to illicit drug use or sexual activity, are difficult to handle sensitively within the format of a self-completion questionnaire or even a face-to-face interviewer-completion survey. This is true of any age group, but is particularly pertinent in dealing with younger adolescents where parental or school consent may be withdrawn if questions are deemed to promote, imply or normalise 'deviant' health behaviours in any way.

Qvortrup (1990) raises another problem which he identifies in many of the aggregated statistics which purport to be about children and young people. Describing his claim as 'a very modest one' he makes the following plea:

No more and no less, it envisages giving a voice to children at the aggregate level, with the purpose of discovering the life conditions of children as a population group. It suggests liberating childhood from the representational straitjackets of conventional statistical categories, which at the moment represent children only indirectly.   (1990: 80)

He goes on to point out that where official statistics are gathered about social phenomena, children are almost always described in accordance with parents' income, mostly father's occupation, with the education of parents, and so on. He comments that this approach is not wrong in itself. It has, nonetheless, a major drawback in relation to a description of children's own life situation; namely that it splits up the population of children according to variables which are alien to their life expressions.

Sgritta and Saporiti (1989) also concur with Qvortrup's feeling that this is a way of depriving children of an account of themselves in their own right and illustrate the point with an analysis of a number of statistical source books where there is a paucity of information about children. Family statistics, in particular, demonstrate the reluctance of the state to snoop on this essentially private sphere.

Shucksmith (1994), for instance, in a review of work on the problems of children living in families where alcohol misuse is a problem, could not derive figures from existing datasets which showed how many children and young people were actually in this position, and the same difficulty has been found in relation to estimating the number of children acting as 'carers' for sick or disabled relatives (Aldridge and Becker, 1993). Qvortrup's plea is for official statistics to count the number of children who experience parental divorce or unemployment, claiming that the traumas which originate in their parents' lives have as big an impact on young people's own health and well-being. Scott *et al.* (1994), in a recent paper, endorse this view.

Qualitative methods

One of the difficulties in developing this section is that the division between studies which look at young people's health beliefs from an 'adultist' perspective and those which attempt to put young people at the centre of their work is not a simple black-and-white one. It is not, for instance, a simple issue of quantitative or survey methodology versus softer qualitative methods, for even in ethnographic studies which encourage young people to express their thoughts about health in their own words, the analysis which has subsequently been placed on their discussions compares their views, implicitly or explicitly, with those of adults. Kalnins *et al.* (1992) and Bibace and Walsh (1980) feel that, while ostensibly using children's voices, many such studies perform their analyses within a Piagetian framework which negates the centrality of the child's position. Dielman *et al.*'s (1992) work is also accused of an *ex post facto* misrepresentation of young people's account by the application of cognitive models (such as the Health Belief Model).

If we see the level of involvement of young people in the expression and interpretation of ideas about their own health as a continuum rather than as a black-and-white issue, then at the most extreme ends we have either the quantitative survey with closed tick-box categories designed by adults with no reference to young people's own use of language, saliences and beliefs and, at the other end, the grounded qualitative interview or ethnographic study carried out and interpreted by young people themselves. Examples of the former are two a penny; examples of the latter somewhat harder to find. The Peer Research Project on drug education recently undertaken by Fast Forward volunteers (Fast Forward, 1994a) may fall into this category (at least that would be its intention), and some of the methodologies developing as forms of community needs assessment (Murray *et al.*, 1994; Cresswell, 1992) also use the subjects themselves as researchers and interpreters of the data. Such processes are complex and involve lengthy periods in the field training people in the community (or the community of interest) in how to gather and report data and so on.

Between these two extremes lies a range of very worthwhile studies using a variety of methods. A number of recent projects have been undertaken successfully with young people, for instance, using qualitative interviews with individuals in the family over a period of time, with the accounts from different individuals used to triangulate the themes which emerge. Interviews are, on the whole, loosely structured and the approach to the data analysis a grounded one, the intention being that the themes that emerge are not simply the researcher's imposed agenda.

Significant problems exist in interviewing young people on a one-to-one basis. In particular Farquhar (1990) has pointed to the lack of development of methods for exploration with young people on health topics, and has rehearsed some of the practical problems as well as the theoretical ones which jeopardise the validity of a great deal of such research.

It is now commonplace, for instance, to reflect on how an imbalance of power in an interview setting may compromise the validity of the account obtained. The problem exists in all research carried out by this method, for the interviewer/ interviewee relationship almost always reflects an asymmetry of power, often exacerbated by a social class differential. With young people, however, this imbalance is particularly acute, since the interview relationship often mimics the usual social relationships between adults and children. Farquhar comments:

> Children will already have direct experience of unequal power relationships with a variety of adults. They will have learnt, through experience, both the explicit and implicit rules which govern adult–child relationships in schools, particularly teacher–child relationships, and will bring this knowledge and experience to bear on their relationships with unfamiliar adults who enter this context. (1990: 23)

A further dimension to this problem is discussed by Backett and Alexander (1991), who note that a particular problem involved in interviewing children comes in disentangling the 'public' and 'private' accounts that children are prepared to give. Many research techniques, for example, encourage children to reproduce the messages that they have absorbed from teachers, from television (Michell and West, 1997) or from other forms of media campaign. Reproduction of such 'public' messages, however, gives us little insight into the 'private' logic and reasoning that guides children's beliefs, values and actions.

A further problem for the interviewer using qualitative methods (which can be falsely masked in other types of research where all the subject has to do is respond to the researcher's categories) is that children's powers of expression may seem to be poor. The problem may lie not with a language deficit but with their ability to be sufficiently metacognitive (Nisbet and Shucksmith, 1986). They are not in the habit, perhaps, of being reflective or thinking about their own thinking. McGurk and Glachan (1988) suggest that the principal problem that young people may have is that they cannot empathise with the interviewer's position sufficiently to understand why or what they might want to tap in the recesses of their thinking.

For these reasons, many researchers have developed innovative interviewing techniques for use with young people, which avoid the directly inquisitorial style of the classic interview (Williams *et al.,* 1989; Backett and Alexander, 1991; Scott *et al.,* 1994). What we clearly have to be aware of is the fact that an apparent inability to express themselves on the subject of health in terms that are useful for us in our studies is not a sign of deficit of intellect or reasoning. Rather it is an inability to find an appropriate register or route through which their own sentiments and reasoning might be expressed, and the thoughtful researcher will struggle hard to provide this for, or negotiate this with, respondents. McGurk and Glachan comment in relation to their own study:

> We were frequently struck by the extent to which our adolescent respondents felt short changed by the adults, including parents and teachers with whom they came into contact . . . these young people were asking of adults that there should be greater reciprocity in their exchanges with them. The young people displayed complex and sophisticated awareness of the psychological and motivational processes underlying adult identity, knowledge and authority. What they seemed to be asking for was a reflection of that maturity in adult representations of adolescence.   (1988: 34)

In summary, then, most of what we know about young people's actual health behaviours rests on large-scale questionnaire surveys, which paint very generalised pictures of young people's behaviour using aggregated statistics. Such data often give us little feel for how particular health behaviours are integrated into young people's lifestyles. Moreover, most official statistics about young people are not only collected on issues which have been identified by adults as important, but are also collected and displayed according to criteria (for example socio-economic status of father) that have little meaning in young people's own lives. Alternative means of exploring behaviour (using, for example, ethnographic accounts of young people's drinking groups or gangs of 'sniffers') give vivid and illuminating accounts of how specific health behaviours are embedded in more general youth cultures, but they are usually small in scope and it is impossible to generalise from them with any confidence. Attempts to penetrate young people's perspectives using more sympathetic, qualitative methods are also fraught with difficulty. The imbalance in the power relationship between any interviewer and interviewee is exacerbated in the case of young people. Sensitive and imaginative techniques are thus required if young people are to be allowed to generate their own agendas about health and discuss them with confidence.

Research design of the study

The study reported here was essentially composed of three parts:

- a desk study reviewing previous work and analysing existing survey data to examine adolescent health issues as now defined by adults;
- a preliminary study using ten group discussions to establish an initial agenda of young people's concerns;
- a major study based around approximately sixty individual qualitative interviews to explore different saliences and priorities.

Material from the desk study is incorporated in chapter 1 and then through the interpretative notes in the remaining chapters. In the following sections we describe the gathering and analysis of the empirical data.

Selecting a sampling framework

The second phase of the work was to be carried out with a cohort of 15-year-olds in focus groups with five to six people in each. Previous research (Hendry *et al.*, 1991) led the research team to propose a division by gender, as they had found mixed groups to need longer lead-in meetings before settling down to relevant discussion, and even after this process many girls remained intimidated by boys' presence in terms of raising issues pertinent to themselves (Lee, 1988). Work with pilot groups at the early stages of the research when no gender segregation was practised bore out these feelings. The research brief had specified the use of both male and female interviewers, so that there could be gender matching between interviewer and interviewee. Some research does suggest that perceived similarity between interviewer and interviewee increases rapport, with certain personal characteristics of the interviewer, such as age and style of dress, also influencing the degree of trust felt by the respondent (Moore and Rosenthal, 1993). The significance of gender identification between interviewer and respondent has long been a feature of note in sociological writings, but McKeganey and Bloor (1991) have recently argued that gender issues may be accorded too much importance in this respect. They argue, first, that the influence of gender may be negotiated with respondents rather than ascribed, and second, that other variables, such as age and social class, may be more important. Silverman (1993) feels that this is not an excuse to 'throw the baby out with the bath water' and ignore gender issues, but rather that we would do well to become conscious that even taken-for-granted assumptions may be culturally and historically specific.

All but one of the group discussions took place in school settings (the exception was made for a boys' group from a school for young people with behavioural difficulties, on staff advice), though in each case the aim (not always achieved) was to hold the discussions privately and in a separate and comfortable setting with no other adult present and with full assurances of confidentiality given to all taking part. Research workers were instructed to establish ground rules for the conduct of the group which would also ensure confidentiality between group members.

At this stage of the project, also, the research team was curious to attempt to determine in a simple way whether there were significant local variations in young people's beliefs and responses. However, the suggested design of the sample in the tender document 'cut the pack' in too many ways in order to incorporate different dimensions of the heterogeneity of youth experience. Some of these were felt to be worth preserving, namely gender, urban–rural, geographical spread within Scotland, social class. Others, it was decided, would need to be sacrificed (principally the school/non-school distinction). There were clearly other dimensions that were entirely neglected yet which might have been significant, for example ethnic differences, religious differences. The sample could clearly not cover all of these.

One of the omissions in the initial draft for the sampling framework, however, did seem significant. It was felt that the school framework for the sample might lead to particularly 'at-risk' groups in health terms being ignored (for example truants, non-attenders, sick children). Another issue noted was the unsatisfactory nature of traditional classifications of young people's social class. Young people's own career trajectories have been shown in research to be more clearly related to health beliefs and actions (Glendinning *et al.*, 1992) than the occupational status of their parents.

In the end the decision was made to adopt a purposive sample along the following lines. A boys' group and a girls' group of 15-year-olds would be chosen from each of five settings, giving ten focus groups in all. Four of the settings were ordinary secondary schools with a comprehensive intake. Thus a rural secondary school was selected in the then Grampian region of Scotland, an inner-city secondary in Strathclyde, a secondary in an affluent suburb of one of Scotland's major cities and a secondary in one of Scotland's New Towns. In addition, a boys' group was taken from a school for children with emotional and behavioural difficulties. Few girls are assigned to this sort of regime, so we sought a matching girls' group among the pupils in a special unit for persistent non-attenders established in a secondary school in the same city.

Within each of these settings there was, of course, the problem of how to contact and select about five young people prepared to sit down and have a group discussion from cold about health issues. Selecting young people unknown to each other might in these circumstances have proved counterproductive, given the time needed with strangers to build up trust, establish a group dynamic and so on. It was decided that a better plan would therefore be for teachers to suggest a single student of each gender according to the specifications laid down by the research assistant in each case. Each student was then to be asked to suggest up to four or five friends with whom they would like to be interviewed. The group was then approached to seek their agreement to take part in the session. In some cases schools required written permission from parents before going ahead.

However, in practice it is clear that despite careful briefing of teachers by the fieldworkers, shortcuts were often taken in schools and the groups which were presented to the fieldworkers as friendship groups were selected on the basis of teachers' knowledge and not by young people themselves.

At the group interview young people were asked if they wished to participate further, and, if they did, were asked to give some details of name and contact numbers so that they could be re-contacted for individual interview. Almost all those involved in the groupwork agreed to be involved in the second phase of fieldwork.

Piloting for the group interviews

Each group interview was planned to last approximately one hour. A formal interview schedule was clearly not appropriate, but an agenda of issues was required. A series of pilot activities at a co-operative city school allowed the research team to explore a variety of groupwork methods informally and then to establish a list of salient issues from young people's own perspectives and in their own vocabulary. A decision was made early in the piloting that, if a true estimate were to be obtained of the extent to which health and health needs figure at all on young people's agenda, the project should not be introduced as a project on 'health', but rather as one concerned generally with exploring young people's thoughts on 'issues which concern them'. Procedures at the first part of the pilot stage were very informal, with a total of about forty young people in two large group sessions simply being asked first to list and then to discuss what they believed young people's main concerns were, as opposed to adults' main concerns. They were also questioned as to which issues within their own family were sources of agreement or disagreement with parents. This stage of the piloting provided a clear picture of the issues which dominated young people's thoughts and lives (in the pilot groups, at least) and allowed the researchers to develop some different techniques for small-group work based on the concerns identified.

In the second stage of pilot testing the school allowed us to work with small, single-sex friendship groups similar to those which would be contacted in the main study. Here the aim was to try out and find the best of a range of possible techniques which would stimulate discussion not just between interviewer and individuals in the group, but which would also stimulate inter-action between individuals in the group. A first attempt to use a format similar to that developed by Kitwood (1980), where individuals were asked to volunteer vignettes about episodes in their life was abandoned as being intimidating and unsuitable for a group format. Instead the researchers returned to the specific concerns identified by young people and turned them into a card game.

Cards were made up detailing specific situations, and confront-ing young people with the question, 'What would you do if . . .?' Topics included such items as: 'What would you do if your mum is told that you are smoking?' 'What would you do if someone suggests that you try inhaling something?' 'What would you do if you suspect one of your friends is not eating properly?' 'What would you do if a friend of yours seems withdrawn and refuses to be cheered up?' Each person in the group in turn had to pick up a card and then answer the question. When they had made an attempt at it others in the group would be encouraged to join in and comment. This method proved successful and popular, and was gradually refined over several sorties in the field, changing wording, re-ordering the sequence in which cards were presented and so on.

It was clear from these early encounters that, though the inten-tion was to standardise the method used by both interviewers, the level and nature of responses by boys and girls to the stimulus materials were quite different, and necessitated quite different types of intervention by the interviewers in order to make young people feel comfortable enough to disclose information. This topic is discussed again later in this section.

Group interviews

Throughout the period of piloting contacts had been made with schools, permission gained from local authorities, headteachers and, in some cases, parents, and interviewing in the main sample schools could now go ahead. Schools were asked to help select the sample of young people at each centre, and were also asked to distribute a small pamphlet prepared by the research team aimed at informing and reassuring young people about the aims of the study.

The format chosen led to a semi-structured agenda for the interviews, but interviewers used their discretion in allowing discussions to develop or in moving the group along to a new card or topic. Group interviews were recorded in all cases and interviews subsequently transcribed and analysed.

Individual interviews

Those who have examined the dynamics of focus-group work point to the so-called 'risky shift' phenomenon (Douglas, 1985) where groups are often more ready to countenance risks than are individuals. Group members, in other words, may encourage each other, provoke each other to a new position. In addition, group members often experience pressure towards consensus and unanimity (Melton *et al.*, 1988), and this effect may be exacerbated in groups of young people. This alone would be justification for triangulating the groupwork with a stage involving individual interviews of the same young people.

The research team believed strongly that the individual interviews with young people should be collaborative in style. Such a method is particularly suited to sensitive topics (Lee, 1993) and to people of this age who are often intimidated by direct questioning when interviewed individually.

A period of further piloting with individual young people at the same co-operative local school in Aberdeen allowed the development of techniques for the individual work. Again the concern was not to 'lead' the interviewee too obviously on to health topics, but to gain an estimate of how salient these were in their lives overall. After piloting a number of different approaches the decision was made to develop a format used in a previous project undertaken by this research unit, namely the Young People's Leisure and Lifestyles Project. The method involved the plotting of life history charts (Hedges, 1981) with young people to explore what were for them the critical points and incidents in their life to date and to use these as anchor points against which they might reconstruct episodes that brought about changes in habits, beliefs or behaviours. What is clearly critical is not the chart itself which is derived from this exercise (these were in fact discarded and not analysed) but rather the potential of the technique for encouraging children to give more than a single-phrase response to an inquiry. In addition it was felt to be important that young people's accounts at this interview related directly to their own situation, rather than to a hypothetical 'What if . . .?' situation, or to an abstract inquiry about young people generally.

The form of the interview arrived at after piloting involved a lifeline chart, encouraging young people to look at themselves five years previously and to reflect on the changes in their lives since then. In addition they were asked to project five years into the future to predict their lifestyle as young adults. Pilot work at a further secondary school with individual 15-year-olds confirmed the utility of the work. In practice, however, the two research workers noted that boys and girls responded quite differently to the format and that they had to adjust the technique in consequence. Girls were very disclosing in this setting and needed little stimulus to expand on their accounts, to raise new topics and so on. Boys, on the other hand, seemed more intimidated by the openness of the format, and it was eventually adjusted for them by inserting more structured questions, albeit using the same general framework.

Altogether forty-four young people were interviewed individually. Each interview lasted approximately one hour. All of the individual interviews were tape recorded and subsequently transcribed. This process was worthwhile and necessary since it was important to conserve both the tone and context of young people's accounts.

Data analysis was shared between the four members of the research team. Fieldworkers identified initial themes that they saw as emerging clearly from the young people's accounts.

Transcriptions were then trawled to gather data on these topics. In discussion within the group other topics were subsequently identified and themes of a more conceptual nature were explored in discussion and then through the data.

We move on to look in the following chapters at the results emerging from this intensive period of data collection.

3 'You look in all these magazines and you see all these supermodels . . .'
Body image, appearance and health

Introduction

In this chapter we look at one of the issues which emerged as a principal concern of the young people in this study, namely appearance and weight, linked to concerns about their attractiveness and popularity. The issue of food and nutrition was rarely seen by these young people as a health concern, though they could quote chapter and verse of the health education they had received at school on the topic, or the lectures from parents about vegetables and brown bread. Instead, their concerns about their food intake were clearly linked to issues of weight and its association with body shape and attractiveness.

We start this chapter by outlining some of the previous work on the topic. This deals with young people's obsession with the topic, seeing it largely as a result of the body changes thrust upon young people by their pubertal bodies and the confluence of this with the consumer culture idealisation of thinness. We then let young people have their say on the topic.

Puberty and 'body image'

There seems little doubt that some of the most important events to which young people have to adjust are the multitude of physiological and bodily changes which occur during early to mid-adolescence and which are associated with what is generally known as puberty. The physiological changes of puberty inevitably exercise a profound effect upon youth. The body alters radically in size and shape, and it is not surprising that many adolescents experience a period of clumsiness as they attempt to adapt to these changes. The body also alters in function, and new and sometimes worrying physical experiences such as the girl's first period, or the boy's nocturnal emissions, have to be understood. Perhaps most important of all, however, is the effect that such physical changes have upon identity. The development of the individual's identity requires not only the notion of being separate and different from others, but also a sense of self-consistency, and a firm knowledge of how one appears to the rest of the world. Dramatic bodily changes seriously affect these aspects of identity, and represent a considerable challenge in adaptation for even the most well-adjusted young person. Simmons and Rosenberg (1975), for instance, have reported studies in which adolescents were asked what they did and did not like about themselves. Results showed that those in early adolescence primarily used physical characteristics to describe themselves, and it was these characteristics which were most often disliked. It was not until later adolescence that intellectual or social aspects of personality were widely used in self-description, but these characteristics were much more frequently liked than disliked. It is, therefore, just at the time of most rapid physical change that appearance is of critical importance for the individual, both for his or her self-esteem as well as for popularity, and this is powerfully reinforced by media images of cultural values of beauty and fitness.

There is increasing concern about the extent to which obsession with 'body image' is noticeable among young people. Refusal to grow up, or rejection of an adult body shape can be reinforced by apparently desirable adult stereotypes. Featherstone (1991) accuses the health education movement of exacerbating this trend, pointing to the British Health Education Council in the 1970s and its use of advertising messages to highlight the cosmetic rewards of fitness and dietary care. Within this logic, as Featherstone points out, fitness and slimness become associated with energy, drive, vitality, but also with worthiness as a person:

likewise the body beautiful comes to be taken as a sign of prudence and prescience in health matters.

(Featherstone, 1991: 183)

The mass media has not been slow to pick up on this trend with many women's magazines and tabloid newspapers running spreads with quizzes, calorie charts, self-help guides and so on. Specialist slimming magazines contribute to the genre. The emphasis throughout is on self-surveillance. Slimness is almost ineradicably associated with good health, despite studies such as those by Bruch (1957) and Beller (1977) that the overweight generally live longer, that the height/weight charts originally developed by insurance companies and now widely used as the basis for calculating ideal 'healthy' weight for each individual are grossly inaccurate and that slimness has little to do with health.

Young people are quick to pick up the message that they need to be slim to live out their version of what Hepworth and Feather-stone have caricatured as the Martini people lifestyle (1982). A publication aimed at young people (*Young Scot*, 1993) pointed out that in a study of 4,000 young people in Scotland, 40 per cent of 15-year-olds said they thought they should lose weight, and half were already on some sort of diet.

Coleman and Hendry (1990) have summarised a host of earlier works demonstrating the social importance of physical attractiveness by pointing out the various effects of adolescents possessing an overweight or underweight physique in certain social contexts. There are adjustment problems for adolescents who possess an 'inadequate physique'. Those who are fat and overweight also experience concerns with self-image and have difficulty in social relationships. Boys and girls who are over-weight are commonly considered less physically attractive and must learn to live with crude witticisms alluding to their obesity. Underweight adolescents can more readily disguise their body type with careful deployment of clothing but still usually feel self-conscious about their slender profiles. Overweight adoles-cents are likely to feel that the body is grotesque or should be regarded with contempt, for, as Featherstone points out:

appearance is taken as a reflex of the self within consumer culture, and the penalties of bodily neglect are a lowering of one's acceptability as a person, as well as an indication of laziness, low self-esteem and even moral failure.

(1991: 186)

Pubertal changes attract the attention of the adolescent to his or her own body because they raise the issue of identity. Adolescents observe changes, evaluate them, attempt to integrate them in a personal 'style' and invite (sometimes even challenge) others, more or less consciously, to be involved in the quest for identity, since identity is not just 'for oneself', but also 'for others' (Goffman, 1971; Rodriguez-Tomé, 1972). 'Body image', therefore, is not a reflection of the body as it is, but is an interpretation of it. These interpretations are influenced by individual factors and by contextual ones such as the meaning and values which the surrounding culture confers on masculine and feminine physiques (Lerner, 1985; Coleman and Hendry, 1990; Bruchon-Schweitzer, 1990).

Adolescents are inevitably confronted, perhaps for the first time, with cultural standards of beauty and attractiveness in relation to evaluating their 'body image'. The influence of these standards may come to the individual directly, for instance, via media images or by the reactions of others (Eagly *et al.*, 1991). Research on 'body image' suggests that adolescent and adult women frequently express dissatisfaction with their body shape and weight (Fallon and Rozin, 1985, in the USA; Tiggemann and Pennington, 1990, in Australia). Many young women in a North American study judged that they were too fat, even when they were in fact of average build or thin. This was particularly true if they came from middle-class or wealthy upper-class backgrounds (Duncan *et al.*, 1985). Adolescent (and adult) men in this study were not subject to the same social pressures (that is, to be slim) unless they were particularly overweight, though many of them would have liked to be more muscular. Nevertheless, with the advent of high-profile male models and dancers young men may also be beginning to be influenced by these cultural images. The concern of young people with their weight is frequently accompanied by dieting practices, and sometimes by serious eating disorders (Greenfield *et al.*, 1987; Ledoux *et al.*, 1991).

Maturation and attractiveness

Stattin and Magnusson (1990) have commented on the effects of maturational timing on young women. Early maturers reported

weight problems and expressed dissatisfaction with their tem-
perament. Early developers also reported more problems in relationships with their parents, especially with mothers and with
adult authority figures such as teachers. Such problems tended to
be initiated by the young women rather than the adults involved.
Expectations held about early maturers as being 'more mature'
may be interpreted with some confusion by such young people.
Timing of maturation was also noted in these studies to be
related to patterns of social relationships. Early developers, for
instance, preferred to associate with other early developers and
late with late. Early maturing girls associated with older boys,
were exposed to sexual experience at a younger age than other
girls and were more likely to have had an abortion during their
teenage years.

Like Stattin and Magnusson, Silbereisen and Noack (1990)
have examined the relationship between maturational timing and
varied aspects of physiological development with young men as
well as young women. Their results suggested that early maturation has different effects on young men and young women. With
young men the effect is more likely to be positive, but for adolescent young women the opposite is true. Early maturing adolescent young women are more likely to associate with older
males, to be unpopular with female age-mates and to use cigarettes and alcohol to excess. Similarly late maturers, both young
men and young women, were likely to be at a disadvantage in
comparison with 'on-time' adolescents in a wide range of areas
of development.

Rodriguez-Tomé and Bariaud (1990) have indicated that as
maturation progresses young women evaluate their physical
attractiveness but not their physical condition more negatively
than young men. Young men's evaluation of their relationships
with young women improves with physical maturation whereas
girls' evaluation of relationships with young men remains more
or less constant throughout the maturational period.

Some adolescents are particularly self-conscious about certain
aspects of their 'shape' and their self-perceptions of their bodies
may be closely related to their leisure pursuits (for example disco
dancing) and relationships with the opposite sex. An extreme
example of this concern about 'body image' may be a refusal

to 'grow up', 'a rejection of femininity'. There has been debate about whether this common pattern of dieting for understandable cosmetic reasons may lead in its most extreme form to anorexia nervosa, or whether this latter condition originates in an altogether more complex set of psychological problems. Certainly most adolescents with anorexia nervosa report initial efforts to control dietary intake not different from others engaging in transient restrictive dieting. Crisp (1980) and Bruch (1985) stated that many develop the 'binge' syndrome of bulimia nervosa, and other authors have reported that half of their bulimic patients also give a history of anorexia (Lacey, 1983; Hsu and Holder, 1986). Further, anorexic young women who are caught up in conflictual and confused family situations, which can include sexual abuse (Palmer *et al.*, 1990), often talk in 'pseudo-psychological' terms about 'something inside which stops me eating', turning some real and highly conflictual problems in family life, into a solely 'internal' conflict.

Emotional and cognitive changes cannot be considered divorced from physical development at any stage of the life course, but particularly not in adolescence. Perhaps as a result of media images and societal role models, teenagers tend to have idealised norms for physical attractiveness, and to feel inadequate if they do not match.

Diet and nutrition

Are these concerns about weight reflected at all in the type of diet young people choose?

Evidence from other studies indicates a very mixed picture in terms of the health of the young nation's diet. Complex studies of the dietary habits of the adult population demonstrate a change in eating trends. Older respondents to such surveys are more likely to eat three meals a day and to have breakfast. Whichelow (1987) reported that in the youngest age group surveyed (18–39 years) over one-third of respondents did not eat breakfast. The most striking differences found were between smokers and non-smokers, however. Smokers were far less likely to eat breakfast despite the fact that they were concentrated in manual occupations where physical effort was involved in their work. The variations in diet by socio-economic class are well known. People in unskilled or semi-skilled occupations are likely to eat less fruit and vegetables, less brown bread and fewer wholemeal products, less meat and more fatty foods like chops. Gender differences are also worth noting, women on the whole eating more fruit, vegetables and salads, more low fat spreads and so on. Although there are regional differences in food consumption and eating patterns, these are relatively small compared to socio-economic, age and gender differences.

The Mayfly study (Balding, 1986) looked in some detail at the nutritional intake of a non-representative sample of school-children, but pointed out the 'fragile' nature of much of the information given. Even when diaries were kept by respondents, quantities were vague (one sandwich, a helping of potatoes) and the methods of preparation unknown. This study was particularly concerned with passing information back to schools to give them an indication of how well nourished their pupils were, so the vast array of data on this subject was re-coded on to a scale based on assumptions about the needs of the pupils. The conclusion was that anyone scoring in the three lower categories was having a 'less than adequate' diet at some point in the day, and schools were concerned at finding a considerable percentage of pupils in this group. When food quantities were averaged out over the day, 2 per cent of boys and 3 per cent of girls were 'starvers', on a minimal diet of only one drink or a single food item at each meal. Twenty-two per cent of boys and 27 per cent of girls were in categories 0 to 2 (demonstrating an existence based on 'snack' items). In terms of the quality and balance of diets, 48 per cent of boys and 39 per cent of girls had a diet assessed as being nutritionally deficient. Over half the girls in the Mayfly study (57 per cent) reported having tried to exert some control over their weight, but only 20 per cent of the boys declared having done so.

A study carried out in Strathclyde (MacIntyre, 1989) is more difficult to use for comparison because of the different nature of the data collection, but some interesting points emerge. While the majority of schoolchildren in that study either went home for lunch or had school meals in one form or another, 14 per cent of young people were going to 'take-aways' or cafés for this meal. Apart from these lunchtime visits, 36 per cent of young people had at least one other meal a week from a take-away, with 10 per cent of the sample having two or three evening meals a week from this source.

Young people talking

So far we have looked at what earlier studies have to tell us about the psycho-social changes associated with puberty, the impact of social norms particularly with respect to appearance and 'shape', and the impact of this, if any, on the diet of young people. This provides a context for looking now at adolescents' own thoughts about diet and weight, about their appearance and the impact of fashion norms.

Weight, dieting and exercise

Concerns about weight are clearly an issue for young people, as their comments reveal. Being fat was more likely to make a girl the subject of ridicule, and girls themselves clearly monitored their weight and shape in discussion with each other, taking up diets or entering upon frenzied keep-fit regimes in order to keep themselves slim. Boys, too, mentioned using exercise to avoid getting fat and to build up muscularity. Most girls were concerned about their weight:

> I worry a bit about health – quite a bit. I'm trying to keep a constant weight, making sure I'm not too overweight. I don't want to look fat and horrible and have people make jokes about me . . . have no one to like me.   (CB, girl)

> [I'm] scared I'm going to get fat.   (TB, girl)

INTERVIEWER: Do you have any health concerns?
LB, girl: Probably getting too fat. 'Cos no girl wants to get too fat and I always worry.

KK, girl: I'm going to start working out at the gym.
INTERVIEWER: What's the reason?
KK, girl: I'm too heavy.
AK, girl: I'm heavy an' all.

I think weight is totally important.   (FG, girl)

I'm not healthy because I'm overweight. I'm trying to do something about that 'cos you see everyone pin thin. Other people can eat what they want and don't put on any weight at all.   (GG, girl)

Fat is a worry. It worries you.   (FG, girl)

I wish my stomach would get thinner because I have quite a fat stomach. I think I've put on a bit of weight recently. I think I probably could do something about it, but och when I think about it I can't be bothered. It used to bother me and I do wish I could lose some weight. I've tried cutting down sweets and I ate more. Sometimes I think I should cut down on chocolate and eat more fruit and stuff. I never do anything about it. I eat all the essentials you need like vegetables. My Mum and Dad are awfully healthy.   (HG, girl)

The girls who do go on a diet have mixed success. JG wants to be thinner. She says the weight went on in the last five years.

O God, where did all this fat come from? It never used to be there or I never noticed it. I used to be able to eat loads of sweets and the only thing that grew were my feet.

                    (JG, girl)

I think I'm healthy. I do a lot of exercising. I watch mostly what I eat because if I eat too much I put on a lot of weight. I'm on a diet at the moment. I would like to come down in weight.   (ST, girl)

GG, on the other hand, with the school nurse's support, was on a diet from Scottish Slimmers.

When I first went on it must have been in February, I saw the nurse and the nurse said to come back so that she could check my weight just to see how I was doing.   (GG, girl)

The nurse also recommended exercise. GG is aware now of why she was gaining excess weight.

I eat different things. Coming home from school, I wasn't

hungry but I would just go and have a couple of biscuits. At school, I'd have chips, beans and something. I wasn't totally hungry. A packet of sandwiches would have done me. It was just greed.   (GG, girl)

She thought the weight had been put on when her body was changing. She is very motivated to lose the weight and the inspiration has been her mother.

My Mum, she's small and she was big. My Mum has lost three stone now and she's thin. I just sit and see the clothes hanging off her and wish I could be like that. Even just losing another stone I'd be happy.   (GG, girl)

Girls very clearly monitor not just their own but other girls' weight and eating habits too. A group discussion in a New Town school revealed that the girls' group could list the usual food intake during the day of nearly every girl in the class, together with various odd habits that they had which might lead one to assume that they were either anorexic or bulimic:

Girl A: I'm not totally healthy because I'm overweight. I'm try-
          ing to do something about that 'cos you see everyone
          pin thin. They can eat what they want and don't put on
          any weight at all.
Girl B: But she [pointing to Girl C] can get depressed being
          totally thin. Do you like being thin?
Girl C: No. I wouldn't want to be fat, but I'd like to be fatter
          than I am. I eat.
Girl B: I'm worried about Joey. There's something wrong with
          her. Every time at lunch she goes over to the toilet [gen-
          eral agreement]. But if she was something like bulimic,
          she would be eating quite a lot and then going to the
          toilet . . . Some days she doesn't eat anything at school.
          We made her eat some sandwiches.
Girl A: She says she goes home and eats a big meal but she
          could say to her mum and dad that she's had something
          at school.

These discussions about weight were carried on not just with reference to each other, but with reference also to images and figures in the world at large. One girl, who considered she had a reasonable body shape, was affected by cultural images:

> I can cope OK with my shape, although seeing all those models at the Clothes Show, I wish I was that tall and that thin.
>
> (KB, girl)

> You look in these magazines and you see all these super-models. You don't see any that are 22 stone! They're all about 7 stone. I mean you don't see any at 9 stone. At 9 stone you can still have a good figure. (FG, girl)

Eating and diet

Our research 'style' did not allow us to collect information from young people in any systematic way about diet, but discussions often led the groups and individuals in that direction. It is clearly the women in the family who are the most likely to try to guide and control young people's food intake:

> INTERVIEWER: Who says to eat healthily?
> KK, girl: My mum.
> AK, girl: Mum.
> DK, girl: Mum and Gran.

Some boys also care about what they eat:

> I watch my diet. I don't eat chocolate or lots of fat. It's important for all young people to be sporty. (AK, boy)

Others don't select what they eat but think they have a healthy diet:

> I'm not bothered about diet. My mum is a good cook and she does great meals. (DA, boy)

> I have a healthy diet. I eat lots of vegetables and don't eat too much of one thing. (SA, boy)

> My mum cooks a lot. She likes good food like pheasant. Food is important, otherwise you get bad health. (GA, boy)

> We don't get too many sweets. My mum buys a certain number

of sweets a week and if they're all gone by the second day, she doesn't buy any more. I suppose most of the food is healthy.

(KB, boy)

One girl admitted to liking fast food and said that her dad who was a chef was always going on at her about 'eating rubbish'! Another girl commented:

I eat pizza mainly and spaghetti bolognaise. I do hardly any exercise. I can't be bothered.   (KT, girl)

Only one boy admitted to eating badly:

I eat too many bad things, though I'm not bothered really.

(GG, boy)

This attitude perhaps sums up the majority feeling. Although there were the anticipated class differentials in terms of attention to the healthy components of diet, for all young people the exercise seems somewhat academic! The impact of poor diet is impossible for them to experience with any real significance at this stage in their lives. Their concern is mainly about quantities of food and then only if they have become alert about their weight and body 'shape'.

Concluding comments

While adolescence is in general a healthy stage of the lifespan, it may nevertheless be the genesis of behaviour patterns which are carried into early adulthood with associated health risks. Because of cultural values in operation in society an important aspect of health in mid-adolescence relates to physical appearance – weight and 'body image' – because the images from wider society reinforce for both sexes the desirability of a well-proportioned though slim body shape. By mid-adolescence young people are still adjusting socially to pubertal developments and are therefore also adjusting to the reactions of others about their changing appearance.

Since our culture emphasises the slim but well-proportioned body shape, young people who are not able to conform to these stereotypic ideals can feel extremely self-conscious and isolated. It is interesting to note that girls seem more concerned about

their appearance in relation to the comments of *friends*, whereas
for boys there was more concern to be attractive to the *opposite sex*.
It is clear that 'unrealistic stereotypes' of the opposite gender in
terms of physique and grooming are still prevalent, particularly
with adolescent boys.

Since sexual identity is very important in adolescence, and
body shape and fashion styles are related to popularity and social
acceptance, these are reinforced by a commercial market which
attempts to mirror adolescent attitudes and sentiments while
providing young people with an expressive field through which
their identity can be projected.

Young people's attempts to approximate to such cultural
ideals can, in many cases, lead to difficulties in social adjustment,
and in some cases lead to serious eating disorders. Although it
may be unrealistic to expect health educators and promoters to
work at a grand societal level in undermining the consumer culture and lobbying for the breaking down of such 'ideal' images,
nevertheless there is a lesson for health education in here. Health
education materials contribute to the reinforcement of messages
about slimness and self-worth, and there is a need for the health
education community to be more reflexive about this rather than
just becoming vaguely anxious at the early age at which children
now become conscious of body image and the need to diet.

4 'Down the Yoker'
The impact of localism on young people's health beliefs and actions

Introduction

In this chapter we take advantage of the structure of the sample in this study to look at the nature and impact of local influences on young people's cultures. Most statistical accounts about young people's health or health beliefs either treat youth as a homogeneous commodity or else disaggregate by obvious structural characteristics such as gender or social class according to the occupation of the head of household (usually the father where a male is present). Ethnographic accounts, on the contrary, tend to focus on small and highly localised youth subcultures, often deviant ones. We have an opportunity in this study to steer a course between these two approaches, not relying on accounts from a single location but not also having a sample aggregated to the point where results are presented as homogeneous across the age cohort.

Bronfenbrenner's (1979) theory of the ecology of human development gives us a systemic perspective on adolescent growth which may be of value here. He looked at the impact of the total psycho-sociocultural milieu on the development and growth of the individual, and saw it as a series of concentric layers. Bø (1995) has built on this, using Bronfenbrenner's two lower levels, the microsystem and the mesosystem, as a framework for his own investigation of the sociocultural environment as a source of growth among 15-year-old boys. The *microsystem* refers to all the primary groups which a person joins and to all the settings in which that individual is involved, such as school, youth club, football team, home. The *mesosystem* comprises interrelations among two or more settings in which the personality participates. Thus a mesosystem can be regarded as a system or string of microsystems. We are asking, plainly, what linkages exist between the different micro worlds that the individual inhabits.

Bø also makes the important point that the mesosystem embraces the physical environments, the contexts and settings within which individuals prove their activities. Bø's study revealed an intricate model of three dimensions, in which time spent with peers and indulging in passive leisure consumption in gangs seemed to be principally associated with non-conforming behaviour. Young people with broad support and friendship networks developed through organised leisure pursuits were most likely to be school achievers.

What is of particular interest in this context is the strength of the locality or neighbourhood variable that emerged in Bø's (1995) analysis. Exploring this further brought Bø to the old categorisation of *gemeinschaft* versus *gesellschaft*. Areas characterised by *gemeinschaft* qualities were stable and had a more long term feel about them. Within these areas people have developed more intimate and supporting relationships, with higher visibility and social control. Areas characterised by *gesellschaft* qualities offered less structure at the informal level, and were less likely to sponsor formal, structured activities for teenagers. People in these latter areas were less likely to invest energy and interest in these areas, believing on the whole that they might move up and out of them before much longer.

This framework of Bronfenbrenner and its extension in the work of Bø gives us the opportunity to comment in this chapter upon issues that young people raised spontaneously and which at first sight appear only marginally relevant to concerns about health. We believe, however, that some of the aspects of more general lifestyles discussed here serve as important contexts in which young people form, share and act out their health beliefs.

In this chapter we start then by examining the importance of 'locality' as a setting within which we can examine the foundations or formulation of young people's health beliefs. We then turn to the empirical data from this study to explore whether there is any justification or evidence for this approach being useful. We do this first by examining the differing patterns of association and activity that young people described to us. Does the way in which leisure is spent, the degree to which activities are controlled by parents, the extent of young people's actual freedom to control their movements have an impact on their health behaviours and beliefs? We move on to examine to what extent the differences in reported behaviour on issues such as smoking, alcohol use and sexual activity differ by catchment and examine whether this is merely a reflection of socio-economic differences.

The importance of locality

Social science writing in the 1950s was dominated by accounts of communities. In the decade that followed such analysis was largely abandoned, not least because of fears that it often led to reified concepts of the community as an active social entity (Gibbon, 1973; Day and Fitton, 1975). This, as Day and Murdoch (1993) comment, led to a 'conservative consensualism' where the interests of groups and individuals were subordinated to those communities to which they were said to belong. Thus accounts played down disagreement, differences or conflicts. Others feared a form of spatial determinism creeping in to explanations for social conduct (Gans, 1962; Pahl, 1966).

Despite this rejection subsequent work has pointed out the folly of throwing the baby out with the bath water and has advocated a return to the development of an 'adequate sensitivity to place, or location, as a significant dimension of social relationships' (Day and Murdoch, 1993: 84).

People's location within particular places in an important aspect of their lived experience – a resource they draw on for particular purposes. It is of genuine significance, and the loss of 'community' as an analytical concept leaves a vacuum in terms of explaining the behaviour and perceptions of social actors.

A plea for the importance of location to be heard and acknowledged is not made without an awareness that the importance of locality as a structural factor in explanation of differences is counterbalanced by the importance of agency. In other words, although we recognise that local conditions (or perceptions of local conditions) will impact on people's beliefs and actions, we are not denying people the possibility of making individual choices. To use a gastronomic metaphor, the 'menu' is not fixed but is rather one which offers choices within courses, at least of a limited nature. To extend the metaphor, few people in a locality will, however, be able to dine *à la carte*!

Reay (1996) looks further at this concept of 'choice' in examining the degree of involvement that parents have in their children's education. In her work Reay argues that issues of choice cannot be adequately conceptualised in isolation from localised issues of history and geography, understandings of the psychological impact of social class and the influences of differential access to social power and material resources. In her study she notes:

> Geography exerted a powerful influence on the options available to mothers and, concomitantly, their choice-making. In order to account for the differences in cultural capital between different social groups, Bourdieu asserts that 'one would have to take account of their distribution in a socially ranked geographical space' (Bourdieu, 1984: 124).   (Reay, 1996: 583)

Exploring this interaction between self-agency and the structural aspects of locality, Day and Murdoch comment:

> In order to understand why locally situated actors adopt particular courses of action we need to be aware of the full range of resources open to them, and the kinds of constraints which they face; some of these will be localised, others will not. But it is important to recognise that for the most part actors perceive these resources and constraints from local 'bases' whether they be the home, the neighbourhood, the community, region or nation. We have to understand how these 'bases' condition/enable action and how they can be transformed by the activities of the relevant actors (individuals, groups, institutions).   (1993: 93)

Work by Callaghan (1992) employs these principles in a study of young people in Sunderland. Callaghan was interested in using the concept of locality to understand young people as active agents creating their lives within a structured context. Following Jenkins (1983) and his study of young people in Belfast, she prefers the term 'localism', defining it as 'restricted spatial horizons':

> This is an important idea, reflecting a relationship between certain young people and their world. It recognises that many young people, particularly from the working-class, do not look to jobs or careers outside their local area.
>
> (Callaghan, 1992: 26)

She disputes with Jenkins his idea that many young people see the external world (beyond their locality) as responsible for any evils that penetrate their locality:

> Localism is about how young people relate to the place they live in, whether they see their future there and the impact of that on their decisions in organising their personal relationships and family life. This does not require that they can't see beyond their local world.
>
> (ibid.)

Work done by Furlong *et al.* (1996) using data from the Scottish Young People's Surveys can be used to look further at this notion about location and the extent to which young people see their future within the area or beyond. Their study undertook the task of developing Roberts' (1968, 1975) earlier work on opportunity structures and labour markets. Furlong *et al.* described the concept of opportunity structure as useful 'insofar as it promotes a greater awareness of the existence of powerful constraints which shape the experiences of social groups' (1996: 552), but they feel the need to develop it to take on board the notion that it is possible to identify

> a set of area attributes which have an effect on transitional outcomes: young people grow up within areas in which different levels and types of opportunities are available, while the social milieux of neighbourhoods may also have an impact on young people's occupational horizons.   (ibid.: 553).

By dint of complex multi-level analysis Furlong *et al.* provide evidence that supports the theory that contextual effects are an important component of occupational aspirations, though the effects are much stronger for males than for females. In particular they argue that it is neighbourhoods rather than labour markets which are important in shaping young people's aspirations. The connection may be both direct and indirect. Furlong *et al.* concur with Garner (1989) in believing that neighbourhoods are not just important because of the direct effect of local deprivation on aspirations, but also because of the indirect effect that neighbourhood deprivation affects school attainment which in turn has a powerful effect on the occupational and educational aspirations of boys and girls. Such neighbourhood effects cannot simply be explained away on socio-economic grounds, as Garner and Raudenbush (1991) have proved.

The deprivation that affects some young people's lives is not just material but also normative. Furlong *et al.* comment:

> As part of the process of socialisation children come to share in the assumptive world of their parents, friends and neigh-bours and adopt similar outlooks on the world around them. Central to these normative orientations is a notion of future socio-economic status. (1996: 562)

We might extend these arguments and say that localism and local opportunity structures also impact on young people's beliefs about health, wellness and their individual agency in respect of their health, as well as on their decisions in terms of health behaviours. In the following sections we start to explore to what extent the young people in the catchments we studied dis-played different beliefs and patterns of behaviour which could be said to be determined by localism.

Patterns of leisure association and activity

This topic emerged as an important one because the pattern of young people's activity outside school is, of course, both symp-tomatic of the subcultural position they inhabit and also strong-ly determines whole patterns of behaviours and interactions. Thus there are very clear differences between the groups and areas in which the young people live in terms of their pursuits and leisure habits. The idea of youth as a homogeneous category is only partially supported by the accounts of young people themselves in this sphere. In this section, therefore, we look at some of the common patterns of activity indulged in by young people.

Shopping was the most commonly mentioned activity across the sample. While the timing of the interview may have affected some of the responses (in one school the girls were shopping for clothes for a school trip) there is no doubt that much time on a Saturday is spent 'shopping'. Often nothing is bought and 'shopping' is clearly a shorthand for cruising streets and malls, meeting and talking to friends. Girls mentioned shopping most frequently, but many of the boys also shop. Often a Saturday involves 'mostly going to town, to the shops to buy stuff' (GB). Two girls describe their Saturdays in town:

> Wander around the shops. Buy stuff; not usually much as I don't have money. Have lunch out, usually at MacDonald's.
>
> (KB, girl)

> I go to the town to the shops. I love shopping for clothes and makeup. I don't buy much but try it on.   (LB, girl)

As one might expect, much of young people's leisure activity is spent in association with friends. Many of the girls, particularly in the working-class catchments, spent their evenings meeting friends and going to a park, wandering around particular areas in the locality and going to friends' houses. They go around in small groups. There are specific places they go:

> We often go down the Yoker. We go round the streets up the Temple.   (DK, girl)

She goes to and hangs about at the flyover at Yoker. This was where she was drinking to celebrate her birthday the weekend prior to the interview. Like many other young people in urban landscapes, she is forced out by over-zealous adult surveillance into the areas and spaces that no one else really wants. Young people in this area usually have a few close friends whom they meet on a regular basis but, on their tour of the local area, will then meet up with others. Thus LK goes around with five or six girls and sometimes their boyfriends. AK goes out with friends. She mentioned three names. DK usually goes out with three good friends, but also goes around in a group of about fifty.

Some of the girls in the more middle-class catchment also had the freedom to hang about:

> We went and sat up in the park at Mosshead. We do it quite often, wander about and then end up there. There's about ten of us at weekends. (KB, girl)

Getting grounded and not being able to go out with friends in this manner is a common punishment and one which is universally disliked. HB was grounded at the time of the interview for drinking:

> I go out with my friends most of the time at nights. But I'm grounded for three weeks just now. I don't want to get grounded again. When I come back from holiday I'm not going to do anything bad. I'm going to be a good wee girl. I'm going to try anyway.

The opportunities for these patterns of 'mooching' and hanging about are clearly restricted for some children by their geographical location, and for many middle-class children by parental pressure to be doing something or going somewhere specific:

> My parents would much rather I went into town and was actually going somewhere rather than standing about and hanging about drinking. My mum and dad would much prefer I was going somewhere. (EB, girl)

At this age some young people are allowed to go into town and others are not. The pattern of permission to do this is clearly gendered. In addition, two major issues for parents in giving permission seemed to be whether young people were going somewhere specific and whether they were going accompanied or not. Visiting cinemas and the ice-skating rink were declared as the most usual reasons for going into town. In the New Town the girls appeared to wander anywhere with or without friends but some girls in the middle class suburb were definitely not allowed to go to the city centre for any purpose:

I'm not allowed. Well, I've never asked to go into town. None of my close friends go so I wouldn't have anyone to go with. I'd quite like to go sometime, but it's all right doing what we do.

(KB, girl)

The girls in the rural area could rarely go to the nearby city at night. Some girls were allowed to go with their friends but not alone. One girl was a bit unhappy about it.

She won't let me go into town by myself. It's all right with friends but by ourselves it's not.   (MA, girl)

Some are allowed to go only to specific venues sanctioned by parents. Some girls in one big city mentioned, for example, a night club which opens for the under-18s till 10 p.m. and then for the over-18s. There is no alcohol available for the younger age group:

We go dancing at weekends sometimes. We're going this Saturday because it's an all-dayer. It starts at 4 and ends at 10 at night.   (LK, girl)

The places chosen by those who visit the city or town centres are far from random, with the selection of sites for display and cruising being done by a set of social rules which appear immensely complex. Young people are by their lack of income, however, prohibited from hanging around in areas where they might be expected to pay for a drink or something to eat. Many are thus forced out into public spaces, especially the shopping malls when the weather is bad, where they are constantly 'moved on' by security guards who see the presence of large groups of young people as threatening.

Despite the impression, given by some, of the frenetic life that young people lead, many of the young people led desultory and fairly inactive lives. The 'hanging about' is perhaps a prime example of this, but several young people expressed a need for the same level of restful activity on their own. One girl spent a great amount of time fishing on her own, another mentioned the need to keep taking the dog out on her own to give herself space and time to think. LG and JA stay in a lot. AA too spent time at home.

I'm quite happy on my own. When I'm at home, I'm on my own quite a lot as my mum goes out at night a lot.

(AA, girl)

Many of the girls, especially, were very family-oriented, and were thus happy for a lot of their activities to be centred around the home and family, caring for pets, visiting elderly relations, baby-sitting for cousins, playing with or helping with younger siblings. The girls in the country area were most likely to describe their activities as lying within this framework.

Sport played a large part in the pattern of activities for some young people. Most girls involved in sporting activities did so on an informal basis, such as going swimming at the local pool or ice skating with friends. But there were girls involved in teams, particularly in the rural area. Two girls played for a tennis team and were being coached. Another girl (KA) who had very sporty parents took part in a wide range of sports. LK played for a football team but gave up because of the attitude of the boys. She goes to dance classes at the community centre, took part in a show and competes for medals. For boys, casual football matches, even at this age, take up leisure time, and several of the boys cycled long distances. Many expressed the thought that sport stops them getting 'fidgety' or stressed, and minor injuries were clearly no deterrent.

Local variations in health behaviours and beliefs

This very general picture can be looked at in another way. Stark contrasts existed between the lifestyles of the boys and girls from different catchments. These were expressed not only in the differences in the pattern of leisure activity or association with friends (as described in the section above) but also in the pattern of health behaviours and beliefs revealed in the accounts, and it is to these that we now turn. Three catchments are selected for the purposes of comparison here, namely the rural area, the middle-class suburb and the New Town. For each we look specifically both at the patterns of leisure association and activity, the degree of control exercised over young people, and the evidence with respect to specific health risk areas (smoking, alcohol use, drug use and sexual activity).

The lives of young people in the country area are circumscribed by problems of transport and access in rural areas and the level of facilities available in local centres. Because they are dependent for the most part on parents transporting them whenever they want to go out, their pattern of leisure activity is supervised and sanctioned by their parents in a way which closely resembles that for the more middle-class children in the sample. One or two of them were allowed to travel into the nearby city on their own, but the cost is fairly prohibitive and return services make it difficult to contemplate such an outing for casual nights out. Only one boy spoke of operating as an independent agent, spending as much of his spare time as he could at the ice skating rink in the city. The consequence of these restrictions is that social lives are conducted at school for the most part, supplemented by long telephone conversations outside school hours. Local sports clubs or facilities provided other opportunities for meeting.

Within the middle-class suburb young people's movements are often circumscribed, not by difficulties of access or transport problems, but by parental insistence that their leisure time be filled in ways which are profitable and organised. The pressure to belong to choirs or orchestras, to attend drama clubs or undertake music tuition was mentioned by many of the young people here. Even where young people were allowed to go into the city centre parents often made it clear that they were happier when they went for a purpose. 'Hanging about' is not a sanctioned activity in this area. Thus, though the group did socialise with friends, their leisure time was frequently supervised, organised and public.

In contrast the New Town group have leisure lives which are carried on almost exclusively away from the public gaze and which are almost entirely unsupervised. Few of this group took part in organised activities; 'hanging about' with friends is a way of life. Complex descriptions were given of the recruitment process for groups, with girls moving from house to house on an estate, spending some time, picking up some more friends and then moving on to the next house where the process would be repeated. Some girls claimed that the group size had been known to go up to fifty-six in this way, although clearly it was usually of less terrifying proportions. Once the group has gathered they move on to a patch of territory that is theirs, either in the park or by the underpass. They congregate in areas where they will not be overseen or moved on. Their leisure lives are clearly hidden from their parents; for some the contact with parents is minimal. A number of girls in this area, asked whether they got on with their parents, replied that the issue didn't really arise. They were, in their own words, 'never in'.

Do such patterns of association have an impact on health beliefs, needs and behaviours? We turn now to look at the evidence with respect to the main health risk areas.

Most young people in the middle-class suburb and in the rural sample lead relatively blameless lives to all intents and purposes. Summarising the findings in the troubled areas of smoking, drinking, drug use and sexual activity we would note that few, if any, of the 15-year-olds in these catchments were sexually active, or seemed to consider it appropriate, given their age. Two girls commented:

EB, girl: A lot of people talk, but not a lot have action. There's lots of talk about sex, but not much pressure to have sex on girls . . . not at this age anyway. If you have had sex you're told you are a slag.

LB, girl: Maybe in 6th year they wouldn't call you a slag for sleeping with someone then because you're 18 and grown up.

Similarly, one of the boys in the suburban setting commented:

It's not really expected of you at this age.   (JB, boy)

The rural girls' group pointed out that certain groups of girls did have a more sexually active lifestyle – the 'casuals' whom they were at great pains to distance themselves from:

The girls who are casuals are like that. They sit and say 'I'm not a virgin any more. Guess who I slept with last night?' Some of it is talk; some of it is true.   (JA, girl)

The boys were clearly seen as less mature in this respect both by themselves, by the girls and by the researchers. A question from the researcher as to whether the casuals who were known to be sexually active were under any pressure from the boys in this respect provoked great mirth from the rural girls:

Girl A: The boys in our year are too scared to even kiss a girl.
Girl B: Boys would feel under more pressure from girls rather than the other way round. They don't really talk about things like that.

Few of the young people in the sample in these areas smoked regularly, though many had tried or been tempted from time to time. Most were disapproving of the habit, seeing it as detrimental to their health and disgusting.

Alcohol misuse was another issue, however. The rural girls and boys were relatively abstemious at this age (they did drink with parents and were able to recount episodes where they'd taken too much with friends and regretted it) and were generally disapproving of drunkenness and bingeing, as the following encounter in the girls' group discussion shows:

Girl A: I don't drink . . . . I don't like it when my older friends who are coming home say they are feeling rough. It's cool to say 'I'm feeling rough.'
Girl B: You're just making a fool of yourself.
Girl A: It's stupid.
Girl C: I wouldn't mind drinking it, but not too much. I don't believe in drinking and making yourself ill. There's no point in that.
Girl D: You say things you regret. It's stupid. I'd hate to be out of control of everything.

On the whole for them the accent was on staying in control, not looking stupid and not doing things that they might later regret. The boys in the middle-class suburban area held a position not dissimilar from this, but the girls in the same catchment were ahead of their male counterparts in acknowledging the temptations of over-indulgence and in being able to recount troubled histories of being picked up by police, being hospitalised or discovered by parents after binges. The chief sanction beyond the obvious sore head was parental disapproval, expressed in terms of 'disappointment'. This, rather than outright sanctions or anger, seemed to be the most common reaction, and one which was deeply felt by the young people concerned, as the following extract from the group discussion with them shows. Responding to a question about their reaction to waking up with a hangover, the girls commented:

KB: Try and hide it. Stay in bed.
CB: Wouldn't tell my parents.
EB: Parents would go mental.
LB: Mine would be really disappointed. [General agreement at this.] Yes, disappointed . . . let down. They wouldn't do anything like dock my pocket money. [More agreement.] Wouldn't ground me. My parents would feel let down.
KB: Guilt trips! Much worse than being shouted at.

Fear of being caught by parents or police weighed heavily upon them, so that though they acknowledged the temptation to experiment, many felt that the risk was not worth it.

Few young people in the catchment were involved in misuse of drugs. Cannabis was known to be easily available, and some had been offered it directly. Cannabis itself was not necessarily regarded as a problem substance, though others recounted stories of brothers deeply in trouble as a consequence of extended use. One young man in the suburban area, clearly living in a very bounded world, touchingly recorded that 'drugs weren't much of a problem for young people in Glasgow' in his opinion.

If we contrast these accounts with a short portrait of young people's opinions on the same issue from the New Town catchment, a very different picture emerges, however. The New Town girls lived in a different world where most were sexually active or, at minimum, very knowing. Losing one's virginity was 'no big deal', and there were many accounts of other girls in the year group who had already had terminations or been shipped down to the Family Planning Clinic for the '72-hour pill'. Sex for these girls was not a glamorous or romantic event in any way. Some spoke of their regret over casual sexual encounters, many acknowledging that these were most likely to happen when they were drunk:

Then I went on holiday and I had sex with this guy and it was a total mistake and then I came back and I wished I hadn't done it. There's nothing special to it. There's nothing to look forward to.   (LiG, girl)

Most such encounters are not planned enough to encourage the use of contraception:

> Three of my friends think they're pregnant. By accident. Most folk don't have protection. For most folk who have sex it's not a planned thing . . . it's just a fumble. That's it. They [girls] all think they [boys] will lose interest if you stop and think about it.   (LG, girl)

If this paints a sad picture of the lives of these 15-year-olds it is probably no more than the truth. The girls, for instance, acknowledged that most of the boys of their own age were probably still virgins, but these same boys, in debating their ideal first date maybe give some idea of the joys in store for a future cohort of 15-year-old girls:

Boy A: Go down the park and have them on the park bench.
Boy B: No, just go out drinking and see what happens.
Boy C: Nah, you don't want to get drunk on your first date. You'd end up in a gutter spewing.
Boy B: You'd like to take them down the town park and show them off, with a bottle of cider . . .

Alcohol clearly plays a large part in the lives of these 15-year-olds in the New Town catchment. But the difference between their use of alcohol and that of the young people in the previously described two areas lies not just in the amount consumed but in their attitude to its consumption and in their parents' attitude to their drinking habits.

Gofton (1990), in an ethnographic study of young drinkers in the northeast of England, felt that what distanced young drinkers from their older counterparts in what is a heavy drinking region anyway is their attitude to drunkenness. Younger drinkers in his study seemed less concerned with staying in control, many deliberately drinking to get drunk.

> Many see alcohol as a major mood-altering drug, and both seek and expect to get drunk in the course of a weekend session. . . . The range of drink consumed, and their manner of

consumption indicates clearly that young drinkers see it this way. Many said they drank 'for strong effect', and that they would choose a drink because of its potency. . . .

(Gofton, 1990: 37)

Gofton looks at the function of drinking in the leisure lives of these two age groups. For the traditional drinkers, leisure-time drinking is almost a celebration of the old working-class values of community, masculinity, social order. For the young drinkers, leisure is seen as transformatory and magical rather than reinforcing an existing lifestyle. Drink, for the young, is a means of making a shift into a world of heightened sensations.

The evidence from Gofton's study, combined with that in this project, perhaps points to this distinction being one which should be made not on the basis of age but rather on social class. The hedonism described by Gofton is mirrored in the New Town catchment, albeit with a different age group from that in Gofton's study. Thus the drinkers in this study are not on the permanent pub crawl that Gofton described. At this stage they have not the money to do so, nor, of course, are they legally entitled to purchase alcohol. Instead their venues are usually the park or the back streets for the boys. Cider is cheap and an older teenager will be bribed or cajoled into buying it for them or else they will prevail upon some of the little corner shop grocers who perhaps are too timid to refuse to serve them.

The girls may drink in the same way when they are going round in a gang with the boys, but they also seem to have access to house parties (usually with older teenagers) where drink is also freely available.

Concluding comments

The point of this section was to highlight the very real differences that exist within the group of all young people of this age in terms of parental control and supervision, of leisure life and association with peers, and the influence this may have on the development of a culture of experimentation in relation to health risk activities. There are clearly major differences in the precocity of young people within the age group, a problem which bedevils health educators, especially in school settings. Such an analysis must help in countering the impact on policy-makers and educationalists of aggregated figures which purport to tell us about the lives of young people.

What have we been trying to say in this chapter? Evidence from the literature and from the data collected in this study would suggest that there are clear structural determinants of young people's health behaviours and risk behaviours. Despite this, young people have agency and can make choices, but the menu of choices is restricted according not just to structural constraints but also to a localised cultural development and norm-setting process. This norm-setting is related to class but also to other features of the mesosystem such as built environment. It is also clear that patterns of housing and planning impact on young people's general behaviour and health behaviour through the provision of leisure space and the policing of activity by other community members. If many young people in working-class areas do not look to jobs or careers outside their local area, nor do they look to developing patterns of health behaviour outside the strong neighbourhood/community norms which exist for them. The current discourse of choice-making in health education becomes somewhat meaningless in the face of this spatial and social determinism.

5 'I don't listen to everything she says . . .'
Family influences on young people's health beliefs

Introduction

It is clear that, despite the emphasis on the development of peer group influences in mid-adolescence, families remain of profound importance in young people's lives, not least in the area of helping to shape and determine their health beliefs and behaviours. In this chapter we explore the family as a microsystem within which young people in our sample were working out their health beliefs, defining their health needs or acting out their health behaviours. Brannen *et al.* comment on the extent to which this dimension has been ignored:

> Most previous academic and policy work on young people's health treats young people as though they are free-floating, autonomous individuals. But most young people do live with families of one kind or another, and it is these contexts that help to shape and explain their health behaviour. Similarly, parents – often contended by politicians and policy-makers to be insufficiently responsible for their young people – do not treat questions of health in isolation from other aspects of their young people's lives. Issues to do with health may be compartmentalised by health professionals, but are part of the complex fabric of everyday life as it is routinely and concretely lived. This is particularly true for young people, whose concerns in accomplishing the transition to adulthood often lead them to focus on the present, rather than on the ways in which their behaviour is likely to impact on their health in the longer term.
>
> (1994: vii)

How much do parents (and family more generally) influence young people's health beliefs and attitudes? It has been problematic for researchers to discover an adequate research design that can answer this question. Lau *et al.* (1990), for instance, used a longitudinal dataset to explore the sources of stability and change in young adults' health beliefs and behaviours concerning drinking, diet, exercise, and wearing seat-belts. Part of the remit for this study was to examine the relative influence of parents and peers on young people's beliefs. The overall conclusion was that parents have a much greater influence on young people's beliefs. The strongest associations, however, were found not between young people's *beliefs* and the *beliefs* of their parents, but between young people's *beliefs* and the *actions* of parents. In other words, the direct modelling of behaviour seems of paramount importance in determining young people's beliefs.

Do such findings smack of determinism? Are young people trapped in patterns set for them by their elders? Lau *et al.* believe that their conclusions support an argument somewhere between the model of enduring family socialisation and the alternative model of lifelong openness. There are clearly 'windows of vulnerability' where young people are more open to influence from their peers, but they conclude 'that modelling of behaviour is the strongest socialisation technique in developing healthy lifestyles, and therefore is the most promising route for public health officials hoping to change those lifestyles' (1990: 257).

Dielman *et al.* (1992), commenting on an earlier smaller-scale survey study, confirm this finding:

> Parental health beliefs are very likely a more distal influence in that they operate via their influence on parental behaviour, more than by direct communication to the child. Parental behaviour is more pervasive and visible on a daily basis, while their beliefs concerning health are seldom communicated verbally.   (1992: 58)

Intensive qualitative studies have attempted to unpack the mechanisms within the family that allow this transmission of values. A study carried out by Backett and colleagues in Edinburgh (Backett and Davison, 1992), for example, focused on a sample of middle-class families, and from 1987 to 1989 an in-depth qualitative study of health was undertaken with them. The main study concentrated on twenty-eight married couples who were interviewed in depth about themselves and their children. In 1989 an ancillary study using the same sample examined what health means to fifty-two children aged between 4 and 12. The sample had been chosen on the assumption that the class of the participants would have rendered them amenable to health education messages and to ideas about healthy lifestyles. While this was indeed found to be the case, these family members had as much difficulty as anyone else in transferring beliefs into actions (Backett and Davison, 1992). Why should this be so? When the researchers explored the rationale for actions (or the lack of them) they discovered a complex web of alternative rationalities based, for instance,

> on an interplay between three sets of common-sense ideas: notions of age, physiological function and risk; cultural norms of responsibility concerning social relationships; and financial and temporal constraints consequent on demographic position (such as being single, becoming parents, having ageing relatives). (1992: 56)

What is clear from this is that parents, for instance, operate with a different set of expectations about what is appropriate behaviour for young people:

> it was evident that behaviours which threatened life and limb (such as dangerous sports, motorbike riding, or driving too fast) might be viewed by respondents as acceptable in the young and unattached, but were seen as inappropriate in an older family man. Equally, while burning the candle at both ends might be seen as life-enhancing or career-promoting in one's youth, it was defined as an undesirable source of stress, and potentially damaging to health, as one grew older. Here, the important point is that it was not the behaviours themselves which might be evaluated as reproachable or unhealthy but rather that they became so in appropriate social contexts. (ibid.)

The authors do not comment on the extent to which these

expectations are gendered, but there is no doubt that parents do operate different rationales for boys' and girls' behaviour in this sphere. Brannen *et al.* (1994) comment in the same vein about parents' expectations with regard to behaviours such as over-indulgence in alcohol. While parents in their study accepted that teenage children would inevitably experiment with drink, and that this might result in occasional problems, young people themselves were infinitely more puritanical on the subject.

What did young people in the study carried out by Backett and colleagues reveal about their health beliefs? The children interviewed in this study were aged between 4 and 12. They felt that it was boring and middle-aged to be overly worried about health and lifestyle. Where they expressed concerns about health, it was usually in an indirect way and related to fitness, appearance, attractiveness or peer group acceptance. Other findings from these studies demonstrate that young people have a very pragmatic approach to health. Thus they do not think of health in abstract terms. Rather they see it in terms of a balance or a trading off. Kalnins *et al.* comment:

> they perceive health in terms of conflict situations in which courses of action are pitted against pressure from family and friends.   (1992: 55)

The resolution of these conflicts is often by means of a series of negotiations with the self:

> They seek out alternative behaviours that are slightly less unhealthy or they deliberately ignore what is healthy by deciding that they will make up for it the next day.   (ibid.)

However, this flawed rationality may be no different from that which operates amongst most adults, as Backett and Davison (1992) point out.

Brannen *et al.*'s study (1994) concluded that amongst the welter of changes faced by young people in adolescence, health became an insignificant factor. Their youth and generally perceived good health and vitality made the thought of illness in later life (as a consequence of current health behaviours) almost unthinkable. As Coffield noted in relation to young people's drinking behaviour, they find it difficult, if not impossible, at the age of 15 to worry about the health of a 50-year-old stranger, that is, 'themselves 35 years in the future' (1992: 2).

Brannen *et al.*'s study also demonstrates the extent to which health issues are bound up in family settings with more general negotiations about control of behaviour and policing of activities. Their data also reveal some of the gendered aspects of young people's beliefs about health, with young women being less likely than young men to feel that they are in control of their own health.

The study currently underway by Scott *et al.* (1994) on behalf of the Health Education Authority also reveals that parents see little sense in forbidding or exhorting their young people on health topics. They understand that health *per se* has little interest to their children. This finding supports Gochman's and Saucier's work, which, from an entirely different empirical base, concluded that 'health as a motive does not play an important part in many children's cognitive worlds' (1982: 51).

In Scott *et al.*'s study parents seem more concerned about young people indulging in risk behaviour than by more general concerns about health. Such findings find echoes in a recent study by Devine (1995) with specific reference to health education in Scottish schools. She used a checklist of topic areas for health education which pupils at various stages of their school career and their parents had to rank in order of importance to them. Education on risk activities such as drug-taking, early sexual behaviour and so on were considered much more of a priority than general education about nutrition, for example. Interestingly, in this same project health professionals in the study areas were asked for their views on whether there were local conditions that might make certain topics more important for schools in these areas; pupils were not.

Scott *et al.* also echo some of Backett's findings in noting how, armed with relatively sophisticated knowledge, young people engage in a set of negotiations about their own health, in which a different level of rationality operates:

Young people were choosing to ignore the messages they heard on diet, exercise, smoking, drinking etc. because the messages

were out of step with their own immediate behavioural goals,
which concerned the here and now – losing weight fast; having
a 'good time', gaining immediate gratification. Health goals
competed with immediate priorities and lost.   (1994: 9)

In the rest of this chapter we look at the empirical evidence
from this project concerning young people and the negotiations
around health that take place within the family setting. In doing
this we start at what might seem a rather strange place, namely
looking at young people's accounts of how they coped with family trauma. These accounts are interesting because of the light
they shed on the ways in which parents and children communicate and offer support to each other. Indirectly they also shed
light on the more general debate about the level of competence
that children demonstrate in relation to their own welfare. Despite talk of empowerment, most health education is predicated
on the understanding that young people are not competent to
look after themselves or make sensible choices, but must be stew-
arded and supervised while they serve their apprenticeship as
proto-adults. As in accounts from other literature on children
who care for disabled parents or the children of alcoholic parents
(see Shucksmith, 1994), we can see in these accounts of young
people overcoming parental marital breakdown that children
often express surprising levels of maturity, empathy and ability to
exercise judgement.

We move from this to explore more generally what the empirical evidence tells us about communications between parents and
children on the issue of health. Is health a battleground on which
a contest for control or independence is fought? Or, more positively, is it a vehicle within which parents can demonstrate their
support and nurture for their offspring in specific and practical
ways? What differences are there within our sample in the ways
that parents express either support or control on health issues?

Young people coping with family trauma

Young people were allowed to define for themselves whether they
felt there had been any traumas or notable events in their short
lives to date. A variety of experiences was mentioned, from

families splitting up, to deaths in the family, major illnesses and the birth of siblings. What was equally clear was that young people's experience of such traumas was far from uniform, however, and not always entirely negative.

In the sample there were six girls and two boys whose parents had split up. The impact on the individual young person's life varied considerably and their stories represent both the positive and negative aspects of changes in family structure. On the negative side there is clearly some trauma associated with being part of a family where the husband–wife relationship is breaking down gradually. For DK, for instance, the separation of her parents was particularly significant. They split up when she was 3, got together again when she was 6, and then split up again after her brother was born some months later. Her mother and father subsequently fought a bitter battle as to who should have custody of the two children:

> It was a mess. My dad said he was taking us away, taking us to Canada. My mum and dad were fighting over custody. Me and my brother were just like rag dolls. So me and my brother went to stay with my nana.   (DK, girl)

For LG the particular circumstances of her mother's departure were very distressing.

> She had an affair and, like, my mum and dad split up and then they got together because she said she had finished with him but she never. Ken, she was still seeing him. And then one day I came in, it was the summer holidays, I was just coming up to high school and my mum wasn't in and she never came home at all. Like, she just went out to her work one morning and she never came back.   (LG, girl)

There is clearly also anxiety where children have been asked to make choices between parents:

> I thought if I chose my mum, then my dad would think I was taking sides, and if I chose my dad, my mum would think that.   (JG, girl)

Unsurprisingly, there is resentment of instances where children feel literally abandoned or unloved by the absent parent. At the

age of 12 when DK was old enough to decide with which parent
she wanted to live she also had to make the decision for her
brother. They lived with her mother after that and, while she had
got on well with her father up to that point, she felt subsequently
that:

> we started to drift away. He just didn't know what to do with
> me. He started being too busy. Didn't have time for me and my
> brother. So me and my brother made sure we didn't have time
> for him.   (DK, girl)

LG feels much resentment of the mother who abandoned the
family. She says she sees her mother occasionally now:

> when she can be bothered to come up. Because she deserted us.
> She moans at me because I hardly 'phone her now. Now you
> know how I felt. . . . I hardly 'phone her because she does my
> head in. She says, 'I'm still your mother, you know, and I want
> to be part of your life', and I just turn round and says to her,
> 'If you wanted to be part of my life you wouldn't have
> disappeared.'   (LG, girl)

There is clearly trauma too in seeing the effect of such break-
downs of family life on other members of the family, such as the
other parent (whom you might normally expect to be strong) or
on siblings, whose lives have been affected by the break.

> My dad stopped eating and, like, when he came home from his
> work, he just went to his bed and stayed there. He was always
> in his bed and he didn't have a social life.   (LG, girl)

For other children the trauma of the break-up is absent,
sometimes because the missing parent was not a functioning
part of the family and seemed to be able to be sloughed off with
very little effort and often with some benefit to the other family
members. AA notes of her father:

> My mum would get annoyed because he wouldn't do work
> when he came home. He used to get a packet of crisps and
> some beer and sit in front of the television. Mum had been at
> work all day as well and she had to do the cooking and
> everything.   (AA, girl)

Gradually the father had withdrawn from family life and when a house was found the females in the house moved, seemingly to everyone's relief.

> We were quite happy to get away. It's a lot nicer environment. My mum didn't like having her friends over because she was embarrassed by my dad who would sit in his bedroom and didn't speak at all and it made her and us unhappy.　(AA, girl)

Similarly, where the split has been relatively amicable, the children involved often appear to have suffered no ill consequences, and have obviously even derived benefit from the situation. The split up of EA's parents, for instance, led her to have meaningful relationships with both her own father and her step-father. She lives with her mother, step-father, her brother and her step-brother. She sees her father and his girlfriend regularly and had just been on holiday to Portugal with him. Her step-father's two children visit every second weekend. The family is a very important part of her life and how she sees the world. There is an impression that EA enjoys the positive aspects of three families, not just one.

A number of children comment on the change in their own role through marital break-up. They become carers of parents as well as of other siblings, taking on a bigger range of domestic tasks than they might formerly have done:

> I looked after my dad as well because he was nae well for a while and I had to cook dinner an' that.　(JG, girl)

Several commented that, far from finding this onerous, they relished the changed relationship and role that this gave them in the family, because it appeared to give them rights and a certain level of freedom too:

> My dad trusted me when my mum left. He let me do more things. He gave me more freedom and space. I thought it was brilliant. I still do.　(LG, girl)

Other young people take on adult roles in ways other than the purely pragmatic or domestic chores. LG, commenting on her relationship with her father, notes that:

> We got a lot closer after that. If he went out at nights and he came home and I was still up, we'd sit and talk. He'd tell me what he'd done. I'd tell him what I'd done.   (LG, girl)

In a slightly more alarming fashion DK also appeared to need to take on an adult role as defender (in her father's absence) of her siblings:

> A girl of 16 battered my brother. Broke all his fingers. I thought, how would she like for her fingers to be broke. So I went and done it to her. She then charged me with assault.
>
>   (DK, girl)

When asked by the interviewer whether she had always acted like this she said:

> Ever since my dad left us.   (DK, girl)

It is perhaps little wonder that children who have adopted such adult roles and earned extra freedom, find it less than easy to cede this when a new adult partner comes along for the parent and the normal adult/child relationship is expected to fall back into place. LG comments that, following the development of a much closer relationship with her father, he subsequently found a new partner:

> Well, he's got someone to talk to. He doesn't need me. So he doesn't talk to me but I don't talk to him either. I just feel awkward talking to him now because of all the things that have happened, like I've been lifted three times. He's caught me drunk three times. He thinks I'm going off the rails. I was truanting a lot.   (LG, girl)

She complains that while he used to give her a lot of freedom he now gives her a hard time. This in turn, in her opinion, exacerbates the situation.

Several young people commented indirectly on the challenging nature of the relationships that confront them in the reconstitution of families and the complex 'step' and 'half' relationships that arise. The usual mix of sibling affection and rivalry is made more complex, and step-sisters appear both as 'brats' who appear to be favoured or as rather useful part-time extensions to the family with whom you can swap clothes. But usual relationships with adults are also altered, especially in respect of the mentoring role of adults. DK, for instance, reflecting on the impact of the separation from her mother for many years clearly sees her own parent as different from other people's mothers. While her mother is 'a lot of fun to be around', she also feels on occasions that her mother is trying to be a sister to her rather than a mother and that 'embarrasses me. She acts like a wee teenager.' EA, on the other hand, feels the very positive influence that her father's new partner has had on her:

> She brought up her son who was 2 on her own until she met my dad. Her son is now 7. She had a full-time job; she kept her son at nursery. She's got a really nice house and she makes her own clothes. She's always immaculate and she's made me realise that you don't need a man in your life to get everything you want. (EA, girl)

Communication with parents

What are young people's relationships with their parents like? Do they communicate on issues that matter? Are young people able to turn to them for advice and support? In this section we start to draw together the evidence from young people's accounts on the role of the family in their lives and their thinking on health.

As the main communicator within the family the mother does appear to be the first line of support and information for many young people, irrespective of their gender. While some mothers are obviously more helpful than others (and some fail dismally or do not attempt communication on any real level) most are seen as approachable and supportive. This is in strong contrast to the way in which fathers are generally viewed:

> My mum told me I can talk to her about things like that [bodily changes]. (LG, girl)

> For personal information I'd talk to my mum. It gets

embarrassing when I talk to my dad. My mum has always got the right answer. I'd talk to my mum before my mates.

(SA, boy)

My mum influences me quite a lot. My dad's really quiet compared to my mum. He hardly says anything.   (MB, girl)

I tell her [Mum] everything. I asked her what she would do [if I got pregnant] and she said she would take me to get rid of it and not tell my dad. I can talk to my mum about things like getting pregnant, boys and things like that. NOT DRINKING, Mum's against that, I talk to Dad about things like that.   (HG, girl)

I don't speak to my mum about things that aren't important. Only if something is important, I speak to her about it.

(KT, girl)

My mother worries but my father doesn't.   (LG, girl)

I'd speak to my mum more, I don't speak to my dad about personal issues. It would be easier if I did, he's not the type to talk to. He just comes in from work and lies about. My mum's easier to talk to.   (ShG, boy)

The shadowy spectre of the father is apparent from the interviewees. Many young people appear not to talk to their fathers much, or they perceive them as functional adults who are there for a purpose (for example, to play football with). Some young people, especially the boys, do confide and receive support from fathers, though this is not the norm.

My new dad is okay – we play football together.   (ShG, boy)

With dad I go to football, but I talk more to mum about personal things.   (RB, boy)

The harder you work the more pressure is put on you. I can talk easily with friends, but not parents. Mum gets the wrong end of the stick. Dad is okay. I'd talk to my dad about personal things but not my friends as they may laugh at me. I've never thought about talking to people at school.

(SG, boy)

I'd always talk to my dad about anything. (BG, boy)

If I had a problem I'd talk to my mum depending on the problem. I might talk to my dad. If it was personal or to do with her I'd go to my dad. Him being a man, he can take it from my side or both together. (GA, boy)

Dad is quieter. He just waits for mum to do it and she will.

(MA, girl)

Where does this absence of fathers from so much interaction with their children stem from? Is it simply the result of division of labour within the house, with mothers being left to do the caring and the talking? Do mothers push fathers out of their children's lives by their own readiness to step into the role of confidante and main support? One child whose mother left home reflects on the changed (if temporary) relationship with her father that this situation brought about:

My dad trusted me when my mum left. He let me do more things. He gave me more freedom and space. I thought it was brilliant, it still is . . . We got a lot closer after that. If he went out at nights and came home and I was still up, we'd sit and talk. I used to be totally close to him, now I don't even speak to him . . . He's got someone to talk to [his fiancée]. He doesn't need me. (LG, girl)

Negotiating support and control

A number of theorists have explored the way in which parents both support and exercise control over their children's behaviour and choices, and this has resulted in various models of parent–child interaction (Noller and Callan, 1991). A seminal contribution to this field has been made by Diana Baumrind (1967; 1968; 1971). Baumrind's work identified two major dimensions underlying parent–child relationships, namely parental acceptance and parental control. Baumrind uses these dimensions of acceptance and control to identify a number of parenting styles which are labelled as 'authoritarian', 'authoritative', and 'permissive'. The authoritarian style involves rigidly enforced rules, allied to low levels of acceptance. The authoritative style, on the other hand, combines reasoned control with support and concern, in that it involves setting firm limits while demonstrating acceptance by explaining the reasons behind policies and by encouraging exchange between parent and child. Research has consistently shown that parental warmth, support, inductive discipline, non-punitive sanctions and consistency in child rearing are all associated with positive developmental outcomes in children (Maccoby and Martin, 1983).

The permissive style, as identified by Baumrind, was associated with low levels of control, but later studies (Maccoby and Martin, 1983) have made an important distinction between 'permissive' parenting, which is associated with acceptance of children's behaviours and attitudes as appropriate, and 'neglectful' parenting where low levels of control are also associated with low levels of acceptance. In studying the effects of three of these styles, Baumrind found that children with authoritative parents were the most autonomous and had greatest self-esteem, whereas those with permissive parents (that is, 'permissive', including 'neglectful') were judged to be the least well developed in these areas, and the children of authoritarian parents occupied an intermediate position.

The relationship between parenting style and psycho-social outcomes for the child may, for instance, tell us much about the ease with which individuals cope with pressures from friends and peers. 'Neglectful' parents or those encouraging autonomy at too early an age appear to put adolescents at risk from peer pressure (Steinberg and Silverberg, 1986). But, equally, too-controlling families may also put children at risk from peer pressures (Burt *et al.*, 1988). Newman and Murray (1983) see parents' use of power as critical to the shaping of adolescent identities, through the influence that this exerts on the individual's willingness to be involved in identity exploration. Coercion rather than inductive methods of parenting, combined with low levels of support, are seen to produce problems of identity formation, externalised moral standards, a susceptibility to peer pressure, and lowered self-confidence and self-esteem. Thus the implications of parenting style for health outcomes and health education are not hard to decipher.

A study reported by Shucksmith *et al.* (1995) would appear to confirm many of these general conclusions for a population much closer to hand. The Young Peoples Leisure and Lifestyle study showed that for Scottish young people in early to middle adolescence, the most common parenting styles would appear to be either a permissive or an authoritative approach. Two less common approaches are authoritarian parenting, and a 'neglect-ful' approach which is associated with families where there are significant relational difficulties. For this latter group, parent–adolescent relationships are characterised by behaviour problems and conflict, low levels of perceived acceptance, support and concern, and by feelings of detachment. The defining character-istic for young people from such families is of poorly functioning parent–adolescent relationships. This is in marked contrast to other young people, where, irrespective of parenting style, relationships with parents were viewed positively.

Turning to the socio-economic circumstances of the family, the study showed that overall there are apparently few differences between social groups. However, neglectful/problem relation-ships were linked to some extent to social disadvantage, where the head of the household is not in paid employment, and 'middle-class' families were marginally more likely to adopt an authoritative rather than an authoritarian approach.

What then are the potential outcomes of the ways in which families function for young people's psycho-social development in adolescence? Authoritative parenting is associated with fewer symptoms of psychological distress, while neglectful parenting (allied to relational problems with parents) is associated with correspondingly raised levels of psychological distress. Young people from permissive and authoritarian homes occupy an intermediate position between these two extremes. Summarising these findings it would appear therefore that parenting which combines high levels of acceptance with appropriate levels of control is perhaps the most 'effective' family environment in early and middle adolescence.

The evidence from this project would seem to add qualitative data which support these general findings. Though the sample was not a representative one it is clear that the majority had positive views about their parents overall. The exceptions, not surprisingly, were the cases where a child had been abandoned by a parent on the breakdown of a marriage. Few young people challenged their parents' authority in any major way, seeming to feel it was an appropriate part of the relationship. The sources of conflict reported were relatively minor, relating to tidying bedrooms, staying out too late and so on, and most young people seemed happy enough within their family groups. Within many family settings young people of this age were clearly learning to negotiate with parents about these rules, and there were many examples, for instance, of the ways in which coming home times in the evening were negotiated.

On other issues, such as smoking and drinking, parental control or censure was very varied. In some families, the pressure not to engage in such activities is strong. For instance SHG (a boy) claimed that his parents would 'ground him' for smoking. Almost all parents will offer children alcohol on what are seen as appropriate family occasions, but few approve of their children hanging about and drinking with the peer group at this age, and episodes of drunkenness had to be hidden from parents.

Control over activities was exercised differently between the groups, with the more middle-class families making sure that young people were occupied for almost all their leisure time with extra lessons, sports activities, or group membership of some kind. In this way their children are never idle, don't hang around, and parents retain control over young people's movements as they must be ferried from activity to activity and their involvement paid for. Many of the middle-class children felt the restriction of this way of life compared to some of their school peers. The lifestyles they describe sound active and full of fun, but several recognised that they were living out their parents' fantasies and chafed under the control exercised over them in this respect. One girl, for instance, describing how her parents pushed her to be musical all the time, confessed that she had stopped taking her guitar lessons a year ago and that her parents had still not been told. She knew there would be trouble when they found out. Another girl, who spent large amounts of time singing in a choir, stated rather plaintively:

> I know my mum and dad won't let me quit 'cos they tell me how lucky I am. (BJ, girl)

MA, a girl, talking about playing the fiddle, said:

> I sort of get pushed into things and then enjoy it after.
> Mum did push me into it. I don't know why they want us to be
> so musical because they weren't that musical themselves.
> Probably because they weren't.

In other families such control can appear to be very lax. Several of the girls, for instance, when asked whether they argued
with parents, responded that they were 'never in', and certainly
when both parents are working (often on shifts) some young
people please themselves, hanging about with whomever they
like and apparently not having their activities overseen in any
way. It would be too simplistic to see these young people as
neglected, however, or the parents as lacking in control over
them. One of the girls who was 'never in' saw her parents only
late in the evening before bedtime, but she comments on their
interaction at that point, for they clearly all met up then,
swapped news of their day and talked over issues before going to
bed.

How supportive do young people feel their parents are? In
some ways, of course, the elements of support and control are
not orthogonal, but perceived by parents *and* children as elements of the same continuum of care. Thus controls and curfews
are often ambiguously described. Young people describe their
parents as supportive in terms of their ability to listen to them
and to help them handle major problems, like bullying at school.
Others simply describe a situation where they feel their parents
are bolstering their self-esteem or identity or giving them the
right to stand up to pressure from other quarters, albeit over
apparently trivial things such as fashion or over major moral
issues. BJ, a girl who is fairly strictly controlled by parents,
acknowledges, for instance, her mother's influence on her
thinking (in respect of fashion):

> My mum was telling me there wasn't any real point trying to
> be like other people because you're yourself, and she's always
> telling my big sister that and then I decided one day she was
> right. I decided to do what I wanted to do.

Later, she comments:

My mum influences a lot what I do. I don't listen to everything she says but quite a lot. I really like my mum. I did the same subjects as she did. I sort of want to do what she does. We're really alike . . .   (BJ, girl)

EB, a girl, asked why she claimed relations with her family were so good, replied:

I just think we're all considerate to each other and know what would upset one of us. I think a lot of people fall out with their parents because they've said they'll do something and they've not. My parents are really reliable. If they say they'll pick you up at a certain time they'll be there and they've never let me down. And I think that's why we've got a lot of trust in each other and we can talk to each other.

Lest this paint too rosy a picture of family life, it should be pointed out that the same girl talks about screaming at her mother frequently in a bad temper, and of her father not taking any cheek from her, but she does a 'lot of things' with her mum and clearly finds the family environment supportive, despite the day-to-day moments of friction.

Other young people seemed less sanguine about the prospect of support from their parents. In some families control was expressed in terms of the withdrawal of support if boundaries were transgressed. LG, a girl who had been worried about a missing period, declared:

I was totally confused and I didn't know who to turn to. I ended up telling my pal when I was drunk. . . . She said we'll go and get a pregnancy test on Saturday. I'm like . . . is it that easy? My dad's already told me that if I come in and say I'm pregnant I'm to continue walking out through the back door.

This last remark illustrates a feature which has already been noted in chapter 4, namely the extent to which these messages about support and control are expressed quite differently in middle-class and working-class catchments. Whereas in most working-class families control was expressed through direct prohibition of activities or through warnings about the dire consequences of actions, many middle-class children clearly felt more strongly controlled by the sense of disappointment that their parents would feel if they failed to live up to standards set for them.

The emphasis in a lot of the talk amongst young people from middle-class families about taking health risks is about opportunities forgone. In contrast in the more working-class families it was also clear that parents exerted control, not through implying what might be lost to young people but by a sort of bargaining process which accepted lower-level risks for the sake of protecting children against risks which were seen as more potent:

> My mum said last night that she would prefer I drank alcohol than take drugs if I had to do one of them.   (LyG, girl)

The appearance of drugs as a threat to young people's well-being has clearly had the curious effect of making alcohol misuse much more acceptable for many parents and their offspring. Parents seem to be almost unanimous in accepting that young people will drink, and that the best way to help them to achieve this in moderation is to initiate them into drinking within controlled and acceptable settings, and to establish parameters within which there are agreed levels, venues and behaviours around alcohol use.

> Yes, but I only do it when my mum and dad is around because they know I'm doing it [drinking] and they let me do it. I wouldn't go out with my friends and do it.   (ST, girl)

> My mum said she wouldn't worry if I was in the house and got drunk but if I was outside with my friends and got drunk, my mum would kill me.   (TG, girl)

No young people expressed similar thoughts about parents bargaining over drugs (though young people have their own rationale). Parents felt their only option was to discourage use completely.

In sum the evidence from this study is not sufficient to tell us whether it is parental health behaviours that have most effect on young people's own health choices. We have only young people's accounts of their parents' actions, and in many cases (particularly with regard to smoking) they seem repelled by certain parental behaviours as much as drawn to them. Unlike Dielman *et al.* (1992) we would conclude that health issues are discussed frequently and openly in most of the families that the young people in this study came from, but like Scott *et al.* (1994) we note that this is especially in relation to topics like sexual activity and alcohol and drug use, which are perceived as high-risk areas. Few young people in the study, for instance, volunteered their parents' views on diet and exercise. It is clear then that health *is* an area in which the complex web of patterns of support and control that comprise parenting are acted out.

It might be worth making a distinction, however, between talk about health issues in the abstract and dilemmas that young people confront personally. Parents use cases in the media or amongst friends to pinpoint issues and talk through their own views on issues with young people in advance of problems being encountered. In this sense they seem to be mapping the territory for young people in advance, establishing boundaries and routes. What there seems to be much less discussion of is actual instances in which young people are lost or have deviated from the route. We have, for instance, far fewer accounts of young people talking through an actual problem that they have encountered (either through over-indulgence in alcohol, drug use or sexual activity) with a parent. These dilemmas seem to be shared more often within the friendship group.

If we are allowed to develop the analogy started above, we can see that having mapped the territory, parents offer a variety of methods of supporting and controlling young people making their way across the landscape. Direct prohibition of certain parts of the landscape exists (particularly with respect to drugs), but beyond this there are clear class differences. Middle-class parents try to keep the young people going either by thoughts of what lies beyond the mountains ahead or by expressing disappointment if they stray from the charted path. Working-class parents seem to concentrate instead on pointing out the lesser of two evils at each stage along the path, while accepting that there will be some straying from the route. Within this context the messages they seem to purvey to young people are about 'balance', as Kalnins *et al.*

(1992) also noted, and about establishing realistic and culturally appropriate goals in terms of health behaviours.

How do these findings equate with more quantitative studies about parenting types and their impact on young people's welfare? The evidence seems to support the assertion in the work of Shucksmith *et al.* (1995) that the majority of parents act in an authoritative (rather than authoritarian) way, characterised by reasoned control with support and concern and involving the setting of firm limits, while demonstrating acceptance by explaining the reasons behind policies and by encouraging exchange between parents and child. Few parents were perceived by their offspring as being authoritarian in the sense that rigid sets of rules were laid down *vis-à-vis* health behaviour without discussion. While some parents clearly seem, to the outside observer at least, to be 'permissive' in terms of young people's health behaviours, the definition of their permissiveness seems to be akin to that used by Maccoby and Martin (1983), that is, it is associated with acceptance of young people's behaviours and attitudes as appropriate. It is not neglectful *per se*, though it would be a matter of judgement as to whether the outcomes for young people in health or general welfare terms would be beneficial.

6 'I sort of get pushed into things'
Peer pressure and young people's beliefs in their own 'agency' with respect to health

Introduction

In this chapter we look at the importance of peers and friends to young people's health beliefs and actions. Because so much of the previous literature has tended to characterise the relationship as one where the individual is subject to intense pressure from group norms in adolescence, we have focused the discussion around an exploration of whether this overt pressure is felt and acknowledged by young people, and whether they feel this pressure strips them of the right to a degree of self-agency in respect of health matters. We thus look in sequence first at the patterns of friendships and group norms amongst the groups under study and look at what young people had to say about them. We then look at the degree to which young people feel they can choose betwen friendship groups and their associated lifestyle. It is clear from this study that young people did believe they had a degree of self-agency, both in terms of selecting their reference group and also in making individual choices about health-related matters, often in resistance to wider group norms. We examine their reflections on this. If young people see themselves as competent to make choices it is important to know on what basis they are informed. What information sources guide them and are felt to be salient? Finally we look at what young people themselves have to say about making choices.

Relations with friends

During adolescence clear changes take place in relationship patterns and social contexts. Greater significance is given to peers as companions, as providers of advice, support and feedback, as models for behaviour and as sources of comparative information concerning personal qualities and skills. Relationships with parents alter in the direction of greater equality and reciprocity (Coleman and Hendry, 1990; Hendry *et al.*, 1993b) and parental authority comes to be seen as an area which is itself open to discussion and negotiation (Youniss and Smollar, 1990) and within which discriminations can be made (Coleman and Coleman, 1984).

However, both types of relationships are of importance for coping successfully with the developmental tasks of adolescence in that both contribute to a positive self-concept. The significance of both types of relationships is supported by research carried out by Palmonari *et al.* (1989). Part of this work involved examining how Italian adolescents use different relationships in order to deal with various types of problem they encounter. A traditional (storm and stress) model would predict a straightforward change from 'reference to parents' to 'reference to peers' as adolescence progresses. In fact, Palmonari *et al.* were able to show that young people act in a selective way. Depending on the type of problem, reference may be made to parents, to peers or to both. Similar findings have been demonstrated in a Dutch study by Meeus (1989) and in a Scottish study by Hendry *et al.* (1993b).

Coleman and Hendry (1990) have proposed that at different times during adolescence particular sorts of relationship patterns come into focus. They suggest that concern about gender role peaks around 13 years. Concerns about acceptance by or rejection from peers are highly important around 15 years, while issues regarding the gaining of independence from parents climb steadily to peak beyond 16 years and then begin to tail off. It seems clear, for example, that the influence of peers peaks in mid-adolescence, and this suggests that young people would be particularly susceptible at this stage to peer group influences of various kinds. This is supported to some extent by a seven-year longitudinal study of lifestyle development (Hendry *et al.*,

1993b) which showed that independence of thought and action began to emerge from mid- to late-adolescence as concerns regarding peer acceptance lessen. The peer group provides the adolescent with comparison references, sends back images of himself or herself and enables him or her to experience new forms of friendship and intimacy (Coleman and Hendry, 1990).

Young people provided many insights into friendship formation. Their accounts are heavily gendered, and possibly skewed by girls' willingness and ability to reflect on and talk about this aspect of their lives. Girls identify proximity as an important factor in the formation of a friendship group, but one which is perhaps overridden by the importance of sharing interests and outlook. Once the group is formed, trust and mutual support are critical.

INTERVIEWER: What brings the group together?
EB, girl: It's really the area they live in. My friends who I'm friendly with just live round the corner.

You have to be able to trust your friends.   (AFG, girl)

I have similar interests to my friends. We help each other out especially in fights.   (ShG, girl)

INTERVIEWER: What prompted you to go into another group?
KB, girl: I started doing different stuff. [My friend] started going with different people. I ended up with different friends. The furthest lives ten minutes away. We like shopping together and they can tell you what's nice and what's not. We go to the cinema together.

I've got friends in the SNO and I would say I was closer to them than I am to anyone in this school.   (JB, boy)

Young people in rural areas experience particular problems in keeping up with friends who are clearly not 'just around the corner', but there are ways around the dilemma, as one of the rural girls demonstrates:

My friends all live quite far away from each other so we're usually on the phone to each other all the time.   (EA, girl)

She makes the challenge of meeting up sound quite exciting.

The only disadvantage of living in the country is that it takes a while to get to your friend's house, but then that's quite fun. On days off about 10 o'clock you phone your friend and tell them to start biking from their house and you start biking from yours and you meet up half-way and take a picnic for the day. You usually end up in the middle of nowhere and can't be bothered biking home and phone my mum to come and pick us up.

EA's house is also used as a base and young people will stay overnight.

For some young people (although not as many as adult commentators might suppose, beguiled as they are by ethnographic accounts of 'youth tribes') it was important for the friendship group not only to be identified by its members but also by the outside world. A rural girls' group ran through a litany of the various shades of meaning attached to the self-presentation of the various friendship groups within their cohort. There are, as we mentioned in chapter 3, the casuals who were described as 'thick' but also 'think it is cool to be thick'. There are 'brainy' casuals who are 'popular'. The 'smellies' or 'heavies' take drugs and wear army jackets and boots. One group described themselves as 'individuals' but there were clearly smaller groupings even within these large groups.

Girls' friendships, as Griffin (1993) pointed out, are intense and long-lasting, providing emotional and practical support, and being exemplified by trust and loyalty. The girls we interviewed enjoyed going round together, 'having a laugh' or a 'right good doss'. Some of the girls were virtually inseparable: they would call for each other on the way to school, walk to school together, and spend the day together as far as possible. Many girls in this study affirmed this perspective:

'Cos like if you're there for your friends they're there for you. My whole life revolves around my pals and what I'm doing at weekends and nights an' that. (LG, girl)

The closeness of girls' friendship groups rests in more than just shared social activity, but is founded instead very much on the sharing of secrets and confidences in a way which marks their friendship out either from the friendships of the boys or the relationships that any of the girls have with boys:

INTERVIEWER: Who are most important, boys or friends?

KG, girl: Friends. Boys, you can get over them. You don't stay with boys, you stay with pals. You'll be pals longer with girls than you'll ever be with boys. You talk to your friends about everything.

KT, girl: I tell Carol a thing and Carol tells me a thing. She's my best chum.

EB, girl: I tell my friends the stuff I don't tell my mum. I tell my mum the stuff I don't tell my friends. I always tell someone.

JB, girl: If you fancy someone, you have to tell someone.

EA, girl: If you fall out with your friends that's the worst thing.

When I've got problems she [best friend] listens to me, advises me. She's funny as well. (HG, girl)

I didn't feel I could tell Jane secrets. I don't trust her that much. I totally trust Jessie. I tell her everything.

(MA, girl)

For some there is no idea of friendships changing.

INTERVIEWER: Do you think you and your friends will stick around here?

LG, girl: I think so. We've already planned to go on holiday to maybe Tenerife when we're 16.

Some girls have friends who are boys. LB does not have a boyfriend but:

I've got friends who are boys. They're at school and you can talk to them and have a laugh.

Boys' friendships, as others have pointed out, tend to be centred around activity, but few of them could be persuaded by us during interviews to expound at any length about friendship. It is clear, however, from discussions with them about their sources of health information, that boys' friendship groups operate on an almost inverse principle from that of girls. Instead of the almost dangerous degree of revelation and sharing that goes on amongst the girls, boys' groups were clearly characterised by a lack of honesty, with boys describing the need to boast about aspects of their life and activity and certainly not to demonstrate weakness or ignorance.

Given that there is such a division between the ways in which boys and girls use the support of friends, one would anticipate some interesting dynamics at the point where girls' close friendship groups start to break up and they move towards the 'courting dyads' more common in late adolescence (Coleman and Hendry, 1990). In fact the age group under study by us was still too young for such dyadic relationships to have really started eroding the more established pattern. Even where girls described 'going out' with boys, for instance, such social encounters were still undertaken most often in large groups, with the boyfriends becoming honorary members of the girls' gang for the occasion, or vice versa.

> You don't go on a date. That's what old people used to do.
> (BB, girl)

> If you're going out with someone you're nae just going out with them. You're in a group. Don't have a one-to-one. It's too expensive. (AB, boy)

> I'm not going out with anybody at present. We all have boyfriends at times. It doesn't interfere with the group at all. It just makes it more fun. There's something more to talk about, have a laugh about at someone's house. (EA, girl)

Starting to go out with boys often shifts girls into consorting with young people from older age groups, because they clearly see themselves as more mature than boys of an equivalent age.

> If you look at the boys in our year, I wouldn't say they had totally matured yet. (GG, girl)

> He never spoke to me for a week. And when he did speak to me, all he said was 'You're daft.' He's still a wee bam. He needs to grow up. (LiG, girl)

There's no boy in our year that I particularly go for.

(JA, girl)

Relationships with boys are often short-term anyway (with one or two exceptions), and for many years do not seriously challenge the importance of the single-sex group. LK reckoned four months was the length of time she usually went out with boys. Girls in one area gave graphic accounts of the local process of 'getting fixed'. It means nothing very serious and no commitment needs to be made.

Getting fixed is just for the day so that you can see what they're like.   (JG, girl)

I don't usually have boyfriends. I get fixed with boys.

(HG, girl)

She doesn't normally fancy anyone. She doesn't take an interest in boys. She does get fixed with boys.   (HG, girl)

Many girls spoke very clearly of the sense in which they valued female friendships over the very casual activity of 'going out' with boys:

My motto is never choose a guy over your pals because there's always another boy but you can't always get another pal.

(LiG, girl)

If my best friend fancied the same person as I did, I probably wouldn't go out with him, cause friends are more important.

(MA, girl)

Your friends like M says are going to be with you all your life but a boyfriend might last a day or a week.   (JA, girl)

When a girl spends time with a boyfriend to the exclusion of her girl friends she becomes the source of many comments.

She's got this boyfriend of eight months and she forgot about her friend.   (JG, girl)

Griffin comments on the resistance and resentment in girls' groups when one girl threatens to break up the group by over-attention to a boyfriend:

Boyfriends eventually take over from girlfriends – girls do not drop their girlfriends without some resistance.

(Griffin, 1988: 51)

I was surprised to find considerable evidence of the kind of resistance illustrated above and, unlike most previous studies, friendships between girls being largely maintained alongside relationships between boys. (ibid.)

Boy–girl relationships were often fraught, as might have been imagined. There was much talk of unrequited 'fancyings' or of brief romances concluded by a demoralising 'slagging' match. The girls and boys had interestingly different perspectives on this. One girl commented:

I did go out with him for a short time but he slagged me . . . called me names . . . the usual things they do. . . .

(HG, girl)

It's male pride. If you split you have to take a rip at the girl. Call girls a 'tart' if they sleep around. (AA, boy)

There was some evidence that girls and boys could have true friendships which were not based around a romantic relationship. One or two girls remarked with surprise that they had only recently begun to see that some of their male contemporaries at school could be 'OK as friends':

I've started speaking to boys as friends and realised that boys and girls could be friends without having boyfriends or girlfriends. They're not as bad as you think. (EA, girl)

From the boys' point of view girls who were friends could often be a good source of support and advice; they were perceived as good listeners in a way that other boys were not.

I spend more time with my girlfriend than I do with my mates. I can talk to my girlfriend about problems. You can't talk to your mates or mum, so I can share them with her.

(SmG, boy)

I can talk to girls about things I wouldn't talk to my mates about, like what's happening in your life and their life. I can talk to a girl better with drink inside me. (BG, boy)

Girls are friends mainly, it's easy to talk to girls. You talk to boys about girls and you talk to girls about anything else. Well you can talk to girls about girls, but you can't say the same things as you could say to a boy ... like you can't say you thought she was really nice to her face unless you are quite confident with her.   (RB, boy)

It's easy to talk to girls. Certain things that you can't talk to girls about ... like girls! ... I spend a lot of time talking about girls!   (TB, boy)

Not all boys agree with this, with some experiencing great shyness and embarrassment at the thought of even talking to girls, let alone sharing intimate thoughts:

I have four girls who are friends and I hang around with them after school. Generally I hang around in a group. I can't talk to girls about personal issues. I only talk to my mates about them.   (CB, boy)

If I'm in a quiet mood I can't talk to girls. I get embarrassed.
                                                           (ShG, boy)

Girls are easy to talk to, but not as easy as boys. I talk to my pals more, I can talk to them about practically everything, except what you've done with a girl.   (GG, boy)

Peer pressure or peer preference?

Friendship groups and peer groups are not the same thing. Young people themselves are clear about the differences. For girls in particular the friendship group provides a supportive environment which can often protect against forces within a broader peer group which are perceived as hostile. Research which stresses the powerful influence of the peer group and portrays it as an inescapable force which sucks young people into misdemeanours is now giving way to a reformulation which lays more stress both on young people's self-agency and on their competence to choose their companions by shared preferences, thus raising or lowering the effects of peer group norms on them (Coggans and McKellar, 1994). Our findings support this notion that young people clearly make choices in the knowledge that participation in different social networks will involve them in different specific behaviours.

> Adolescents co-ordinate their choice of friends and their behaviours so as to maximise congruency ... if ... the friend's attitude or behaviour is incongruent ... the adolescent will either break off the friendship and seek another friend or will keep the friend and modify his own behaviour.
>
> (Kandel, 1978: 430)

GC, for instance, regrets the difficulty in making friends but also knows that she does not want to get involved in particular behaviour, so she stays away from particular people.

> I think I would be scared if I got into a wrong crowd and then I would keep on doing the same thing and get more and more punishment. I'm quite well behaved. I wouldn't want to ruin that and I've still got a whole career in front of me to get through. (GG, girl)

It also seems that individuals are aware of what would happen if you chose particular friends.

> If you hang about with friends that are older and on the streets then there would be a lot of pressure. I do hang around the streets, I do hang around the streets, I just cause trouble usually in a big gang. Chapping on doors and that. I do it for risk. I like risky things. (RK, boy)

> I don't drink. I'm not allowed to go out at night. Not much anyway. People who go out at night get drunk, but because I don't go out at night I don't get drunk. (JB, girl)

> If all my mates started smoking, drinking or taking drugs I suppose I'd have to re-think. (RK, boy)

Most young people choose their friends, rather than these friends pressurising individuals into behaviour they do not really want to engage in. All the young people we spoke to recognised groups who are into drugs, for instance. Most adolescents would not be ignorant of likely outcomes if they joined a particular group.

I'd get new friends if they got into it [drugs].   (BB, girl)

However, young people themselves talked a great deal not about particular pressures from individuals, but about general group norms and the effect on them in relation to certain aspects of health behaviour.

Self-identity and self-agency

It is easy to get the impression from the way in which survey studies are analysed and reported that health status and health behaviours are determined solely by structural factors such as class and gender. In this study the qualitative data gives us scope to look instead at the evidence for young people's own agency in the matter of their health. We have already seen in the last section the extent to which young people seem to make choices about friendship groups within the broader nexus of the peer group. We continue to explore the idea of young people acting as competent actors in determining their own health in this section.

According to person–environment 'fit' theory (Eccles and Midgley, 1989), behaviour, motivation, and health are influenced by the 'goodness of fit' between the characteristics individuals bring to their social environments and the characteristics of these social environments. Coffield *et al.*'s (1986) model reminds us of the broader social and cultural factors which impact on the transition to adulthood in the various developmental domains; while Lerner (1985) stresses the dynamic interactions in the socialisation process, whereby the individual can be an 'active agent' in his/her own development and can be provided (to some extent) with a personal 'locus of control'. Young people *do* play an active role in choosing and shaping the contexts in which they operate and develop and in their activities and lifestyles.

Lerner (1985) draws attention to the adolescent in three modes: as *stimulus* (eliciting different reactions from the social environment); as *processor*, in making sense of the behaviour of others; and as *agent*, *shaper* and *selector*, by doing things, making choices and influencing events. These ideas concerning reciprocal influences and individual young people as 'active agents' in their own transitional process from childhood to adulthood are important themes in gaining an understanding of young people's decisions about health in mid-adolescence.

Clearly entry into a new phase of the life course challenges self-identity and particularly individual self-evaluations as young people attempt new tasks in which they can succeed or fail, as they alter their values and the areas which are important for overall self-esteem, and as they confront new significant others against whom they rate themselves and about whose judgements they care. Young people's social competence appears to be related to self-esteem and gender identity. Using a sample of young people aged 12 to 18 years Streitmatter (1985) examined differences in identity perceptions across age groups. The results of her study revealed indirect support for Erikson's (1968) speculations about the search for identity in adolescence. The pattern found by Streitmatter indicated that male and female gender identification prior to adolescence was fairly distinct. Entry into adolescence seemed to cloud the issue. The pattern indicated decreasing differentiation from 12 and 13 to 14 years and from 14 to 15 years. However, 15- to 16-year-old comparisons reflected increasing differentiation. Apparently gender identifications which are adopted in childhood are reconsidered and reformulated during adolescence. Gilligan (1990) contended that as girls enter adolescence they seriously confront the disadvantages of their gender and suffer from an initial lack of confidence and confused sense of identity. A second watershed appears to be the transition from school to work if, and when, girls discover how limited their occupational prospects are in contrast to boys. Despite perhaps having achieved better grades at school they begin to have to make hard choices about career and personal life. This is not to suggest that boys have greater powers of self-agency in adolescence: high self-esteem does not preclude irresponsible behaviour. Simply, we should remember that individual differences will operate within the various socio-cultural settings in which young people find themselves.

Work carried out by Gochman (1971) took account of the saliences, perceptions of vulnerability and health motivators of young people. A mix of questionnaires and picture stimuli was used by the researchers on large samples of children, and a model developed linking salience, vulnerability, health motivation and potential health behaviour. One of the principal findings amongst children was of a personality characteristic of perceived vulnerability to health problems (Gochman, 1971), but the author himself warned that the relationship to actual behaviour was not a simple one. Kalnins and Love comment on the reasons for this:

> First, health as a motive does not play a prominent part in many children's cognitive worlds. Second, perceived vulnerability to a health problem was generally not very high. The implications of these findings is that the number of children who perceive themselves as vulnerable, and whom health educators might pick as a logical target for education, is small. Third Gochman has demonstrated that the relationship between perceived vulnerability and the potential health behaviour is mediated by locus of control and the degree to which children perceive health as salient, as well as the child's age, sex and socio-economic status.   (1982: 16)

Kalnins and Love (1982) identify Gochman's work as operating within the paradigm of expectancy theory. They note that this theory proposes that an individual will take a certain action based on his/her subjective estimates of whether the action will achieve a particular desired outcome. We might choose to formulate this as the familiar Health Belief Model. Briefly, according to this theory a person will take action depending on perceived susceptibility (vulnerability) to a particular problem, perceived seriousness of the problem, belief that benefits of the action will outweigh the costs, exposure to cues for action, and barriers which might exist to hamper recommended action.

Kegeles and Lund (1982) give an example of how this might work with an adolescent population in the particular field of oral health. They offer a testing of the Health Belief Model through an action trial that pre-tested children's levels of 'susceptibility', their beliefs and understandings about the seriousness of the problem and the negative and positive outcomes of following a programme of dental care, and then contrasting this with children's actual behaviour. They found little connection between prior beliefs and subsequent actions, and conclude pessimistically that there is little to be gained from educational work which seeks to change beliefs.

Mayall's (1994) study reveals that children as young as 5 years old 'view themselves as health care actors, with relevant knowledge and experience' (1994: 171). They also realise in a surprisingly sophisticated way that health is about negotiation, and they daily tread between the two worlds of home and school, perceiving and reflecting on the contradictions in the messages (explicit and implicit) given out by the two, but with little or no opportunity to explore publicly the dilemmas thus created. A simple illustration given by Mayall is that of tooth brushing, where the messages that the school teaches are about the importance of tooth brushing after meals, yet it is clearly not convenient for the school to arrange for such facilities and the staffing necessary to be on hand after school lunches. Thus children receive an early lesson in the difference between rationality and reasonableness in the everyday negotiations about health that Backett and Davison also (1992) identified.

So far then we have argued that young people exert a degree of self-agency and locus of control in timing (to some extent) their own development and in dealing with issues and concerns within the process of transition to adulthood. This strategy enables young people to cope with particular psycho-social issues across adolescence. Such ideas raise questions about ways in which young people make decisions about health concerns, what their important sources of information are, and how they deal with personal illness. We look now at evidence from our interviews with adolescents about the extent to which young people feel they have responsibility for their health and have competence to make decisions for themselves.

Sources of information

If young people are to be agents in their own health and to make informed choices, they must clearly be capable of accessing information. What sources did the young people we interviewed find the most helpful? We have looked in previous chapters at the exchanges and interactions between friends and young people and between parents and young people. In this section we look briefly at that other main source of information about health, the school, before going on to look at other ways in which young people might access advice or help.

There are clear differences in the extent to which young people respond to the school environment generally. Social class differences have classically been identified in the population, with those in higher socio-economic groups being most likely to identify positively with the school. Recent research (Shucksmith *et al.*, 1995) has also demonstrated clear links between parenting and school integration, irrespective of the wider family context. Thus in this study young people with authoritative parents were more positive in their assessments of school, whereas young people from families where there were clear problem relationships were more likely to be disaffected with school. For this latter group, negative attitudes towards school therefore mirrored negative attitudes towards parents, which suggests that these young people were not only disengaged from the family context, but also poorly integrated into the school context. It is also worth noting that authoritative parenting was more likely than authoritarian parenting to be linked to positive attitudes to school, while there appeared to be few differences between authoritarian and permissive parenting in terms of school attitude.

How are these general findings seen to be of relevance to health education? From the empirical work undertaken for this study it was clear that there were predictable differences between the catchments in terms of young people's response to school generally, and these seem to have carried through into specific responses to school health education.

Few of the young people interviewed seemed to be convinced that school was the place to look for support and information on health issues that were troubling them or on which they needed advice. Much of this reluctance was rooted in poor sets of interpersonal relationships with teachers. Even in the middle-class suburban area, where attitudes to school were generally positive, there was a feeling that school was an inappropriate place to work out personal or difficult health issues:

No one supports us. I wouldn't talk to teachers about problems. A guidance teacher doesn't seem the kind of person to talk to. There should be someone at school to talk to. It's embarrassing talking to a teacher about personal problems. We should have a school counselling service.   (CB, boy)

In some of the other areas disaffection with school generally was clearly expressed through attitudes to PSE and health education, with young people expressing many of the caricatured attitudes symptomatic of trench warfare between pupil and teacher:

Teachers should make you feel comfortable. (GG, boy)

Teachers are smart arses. I'm fed up at getting bossed about. I'd ask pupils what they wanted. (BG, boy)

I hate this school – it's a dump and I hate the teachers. Half the teachers swear at this school – stand and swear at you – and you're meant to take it! (KT, girl)

My dad tells me to be quiet when I get home, and I never shut up, but it's because I know them and I know what they'll say to me if they are fed up with me speaking, but you never know what a teacher would do. A teacher would probably give you a punishment exercise. So you don't know what they're going to say to you, and that's why I'm quiet in class. I'm scared of what they'll say to me. (GG, girl)

One might suppose that personal and social education classes with their non-examined curricula, with the plethora of new resources available for schools and with staff trained in a different range of teaching approaches might escape this opprobrium, but this did not appear to be the case. Frequently voiced complaints were that these lessons utilise outdated material which bears little relationship to 'real life'. The guidance teachers who take the sessions are criticised for not giving enough time for discussion, or for dodging whole issues:

It's ridiculous ... the videos are made in the 70s ... it's changed so much ... they don't get the message across ... You laugh at the video and don't listen to the message. ... [You should] bring the videos up to date and bring teachers into the discussion instead of filling in forms. ... There's no discussion in classes ... just videos. ... Not all PSE teachers are approachable as they just play videos. (SmG, boy)

Load of rubbish, just watch telly. If I had my way we'd have group talks. The videos are different from reality. If we split up the boys an' girls it would be really good.   (ShG, boy)

They dinnae tackle subjects well, just slap on a forty-year-old video . . . crap. They should get a teacher to show us what it's about.   (GG, boy)

HIV and AIDS comes up in PSE . . . the guidance teacher is about 90 years old and gets embarrassed and is useless.

(KA, girl)

We had some Personal and Social Education, this year. The teacher wouldn't talk about things like sex, so you have to learn about it by word of mouth.   (GG, boy)

We get Personal and Social Education; mostly stuff about school, like how to relax. We haven't spoken about AIDS yet. . . . In Primary 7 we got a talk on growing up . . . the girls got it, the boys didn't. The boys had a video on keeping clean, so they wouldn't feel left out. I think we should have sex education in primary school.   (FB, girl)

Well we had a talk in Primary 7 [on the menarche] and I thought that made it clear, but it didn't, 'cos I think I was a bit stupid. . . . I thought that it came and went away. Like it came one day and went away and came back five days later. And then I got dead confused when it didn't. . . . I didn't know it came through the night, I suppose the talk didn't explain much of what happened. It just said you get periods and that's it!   (MG, girl)

In answer to the question as to how this state of affairs could be improved, it was clear that most young people were voting for teaching/learning methods that were more interactive, and for the presentation of information that was based in the context of their own lives:

It should be more social, talking about AIDS, drugs and stuff, more education and stuff. They tend to skim over, never elaborate.   (RB, boy)

(PSE is) USELESS!!! [They] ram down your throat ideas of don't take drugs etc. without explaining the pros and cons. I'd put more input from pupils, hold studies like these [the interview]. The best idea is to give people all the information available and let them draw their own conclusions. We know everything they tell us already. The content is what I already know, it's just 'DON'T DO THIS', and 'DON'T DO THAT'. I pay more attention to my parents. (SG, boy)

Such entirely negative representations of education must be disheartening to staff who have spent considerable time and energy in developing and delivering courses, and we have acknowledged elsewhere the very real structural problems which confront staff in presenting sensitive material to young people on health issues (Hendry *et al.*, 1991; Shucksmith and Philip, 1994). That having been said, we clearly cannot rely on schools (as they currently operate at least) being appropriate places for the whole, or even most, of young people's health education. Too few opportunities seem to exist at present in such settings for the discussion and working through of the genuine dilemmas over health that young people face.

The perceived sources of information (beyond peers, parents and teachers) open to young people about health concerns would appear to be limited, though magazines and TV are regularly mentioned. It should be stated that this is mainly associated with girls but not boys, who appear to rely on a 'word of mouth' system for their information.

You find out about it from friends, from other people or TV. It's all you've got. (DB, boy)

I'd ask friends, if they didn't know I'd ask my sister. She talks to me. . . . She's older so she knows. (FB, boy)

I do sometimes [worry about AIDS and cancer]. If we're watching a programme about it, I'll have a think about it afterwards. It's worrying. (FB, girl)

The problem with such reliance being placed on magazines and TV programmes to supplement inadequate formal education is that TV accounts in soaps and films tend to go for the big stories that catch attention, and there is a danger that young people begin to believe that the situation thus depicted is the norm. Michell and West's paper (1997) looking at young people's accounts of their initiation into smoking gives an indication of the power of programmes such as 'Grange Hill' on young people's imagination, and illustrates well how public accounts become private accounts.

Considerable controversy has also raged in the media recently about the impact of young women's magazines on behaviour and morals. Do such publications merely reflect or positively lead public opinion on matters relating to sexual behaviour, drug use and so on? A girl in this study, talking about women's magazines, casts some doubt on the veracity of some of the real-life accounts being submitted to such journals:

INTERVIEWER: What is it about the magazines you don't like?
A: Boring. All those interviews with people. 'How is your boyfriend at having sex?' I don't know, I haven't had sex. My sister sits and writes in answers, and she's never had it. She's never had a boyfriend. She just makes up a pile of answers . . .

Making choices

In the light of what thus seems fairly inadequate information at times, do young people in mid-adolescence have the information, the metacognitive insights and the interpersonal skills to arrive at their own decisions and make their own choices about health concerns?

Young people were well aware of the difficulty of expressing a view that was counter to that in the peer group. JB, for example, expresses some of the difficulties in being your own person and resisting peer norms:

I'm sitting at the back of the bus where my friends are. They're all smoking and it gets really cloudy and you feel sick but you can't stop them doing it.   (JB, girl)

But a prevailing motif in young people's accounts was the

importance of allowing other people to make their own choices. It was not felt to be appropriate to interfere with others or to tell them what to do, fear of the power of the mob being mixed, one feels with some notions of people's freedom and liberty to go to the devil in whichever way they please:

> I've stood and watched my friends do it and I don't want to do it myself. (GG, girl)

> People who do it, it's their choice. I'm not going to stop them. (MA, girl)

> I say, 'I hate smoking. Keep it away from me but do it if you want. But just don't blow smoke in my face.' (EB, girl)

> Only one girl in our group doesn't smoke and doesn't drink. We don't say 'take it'. We leave her alone. (SB, girl)

When it comes to health choices, girls' statements revealed a greater independence of viewpoint. Girls were more firmly of the opinion that the choice was theirs:

> It's up to yerself what you want to do with your own body. (KG, girl)

> I'm not worried what other people think. I only worry about what I think. (GG, girl)

Boys were less clear, and obviously felt more pressure from the peer group to keep up a macho appearance:

> It's uncomfortable for boys to be asked [if they are virgins], especially by girls. I usually lie. (BG, boy)

> Alcohol ... most people drink every Saturday, but I've never been bothered. My parents give me it occasionally, but I don't really like it. Most times one person drinks, another person copies and the rest of the group feel they have to do it as well. Most people drink like that. Very few do it 'cos they want to do it. Yeah, if one of my mates started drinking, the pressure would then be on me, but I don't think I'd start unless I was two or three years older.... I'll be drinking if I want to.... It's hard to think how it will affect you in five years' time, but drugs can affect you now. (JG, boy)

I've drunk, but I don't do it any more, there's no thrill in it. You just wake up with a sore head in the morning. My parents give me shandy on special occasions, which is boring. . . . I've never tried smoking, it's a waste of money and you are wasting your life as well. You are killing yourself slowly. . . . Never tried drugs. I know a lot of people take them. Smoking and drinking is no big thing to me. If all my mates started smoking, drinking or taking drugs I suppose I'd have to rethink.   (FG, boy)

I don't get that much pressure from my mates. All my friends are virgins. If one lost it the pressure wouldn't be on me.

(AK, boy)

Young people use a number of means of rationalising their choices where these run counter to group norms. One of these is the notion of developmental 'readiness':

Out of all the girls, I'm the only virgin because I am the only one who has always said, I'm not ready to have sex yet and my boyfriend knows that. I thought he would pressure me because he is 17 but he hasn't. But they all jumped into beds with their boyfriends but I wouldn't do this. They [the group] all know I'm not ready to have sex yet. None of the other girls were ready but they all did to keep their boyfriends happy, because they didn't want to lose their boyfriends. I've worked this out for myself. My friends get embarrassed easily and don't like to say no.   (SB, girl)

I don't smoke, drink or do drugs. Most of them here do them. Everyone wants you to smoke. Me and my sister made a pact at 10 that we'd never smoke. The only drugs I've tried are paracetamol and caffeine. I've had wine but I didn't like the taste. I've also had some of my dad's whisky, it was disgusting. . . . I must have been 7 or 8. I might drink when I am older. I'll be drinking at 20.   (FG, girl)

Another tactic used by young people was to try to achieve some balance. If you could look 'cool' in one area, then the group might let you off the hook in another:

Some people want to be healthy and not do drugs. So being

healthy is cool. To others being unhealthy is cool, it's a balance you have to find yourself. I don't smoke but I drink, it's a balance. (FB, boy)

Young people when interviewed provided many examples of times when they had made decisions for themselves and were pleased with their stance, even if the decision might have been a 'wrong' one in health terms. Getting involved in sexual activities provides an example of one girl's self-agency developing. She has learned something positive out of a negative and dangerous escapade:

Everyone says use a condom. You've not got time to think about it. The thing is I didn't want it but I didn't want to say no. We just got on with it. They don't ask you 'Would you like to have sex tonight? I'll use a condom for you.' It would just put you off. (LiG, girl)

As a result this girl (at the time) thought she was pregnant. She vows that things are going to be different next time, though she is aware that certain conditions and settings make decision making more problematic:

INTERVIEWER: Has this experience changed anything for you?
LiG, girl: Yeh, if I'm going to have sex again, I'm going to use a condom. It's got to be done. 'Cos you can catch all these diseases as well.
INTERVIEWER: Do you think this is realistic?
LiG, girl: Yes if I'm not drunk.
INTERVIEWER: Does drinking make you less careful?
LiG, girl: Yes, I just don't give a toss when I'm drunk. Like if someone wanted to have sex with me now and I was drunk I would be able to do that now.

Similarly for this boy, early experimentation has led to re-evaluation and learning:

The people I go out with on Friday . . . everyone drinks. I used to but I don't like it. I used to smoke hash, but not now. Between 12 to 13 years, I drunk often in that year. I smoked hash but I just stopped it, stopped everything. I was getting so used to it, it wasn't having so much an effect, waste of money. I thought what a waste of money, so now I spend it on clothes.

(MG, boy)

A process of learning takes place: Young people want to try things out in social settings. They see it as important to learn from other adolescents and to develop an awareness of how far one can go in certain behaviours and contexts.

In discussing drug usage amongst young people, Coggans and McKellar (1994) stress that what is often described as 'peer pressure' is more appropriately interpreted as 'peer preference'. They went on to suggest that if the active role of the individual drug user is ignored then the role of peers, and the nature of interactions between individuals and peers, will not be properly explained. Thus for adolescents who experience health education but go on to engage in risky health behaviours their motivation will have nothing to do with inability to resist peer pressure or with psychological pathologies. While direct messages about the avoidance of risk behaviours will always be necessary, there is a need to clarify what these messages should be and how best to deliver the most useful combination of personal development and effective learning of knowledge and skills to ensure personal competence in the face of risks such as alcohol and other drugs, as well as the many other potentially dangerous behaviours young people may be encouraged to engage in.

Concluding comments

In this chapter we have considered the role of the peer group and self-agency in young people's health concerns. While risk-taking is a feature of society throughout the lifespan, adolescents may be particularly prone to take health risks through a variety of social, situational and personal factors. Davies and Coggans (1991) stated that we should stop thinking of health problems as features of personal inadequacy or social deprivation or of peer group pressure. As Coggans and McKellar (1994) have stressed, it is important to reassert the role of the individual in his or her own development. Issues of choice and motivation have to be taken into account in health education programmes. Health education also needs to pay heed to the dynamic and reciprocal relationship and interactions between individuals and peers. We have seen from young people's comments how they can conduct themselves with a sense of self-agency in certain contexts and yet feel particularly dependent and require the support of friends and influence of peers in others. Such issues stress the important interactions among individual personality, motivation, self-agency, and the adolescent's selection of friends with wider peer networks.

These interactions constitute the framework within which young people develop socially and make health choices. Our interviews with adolescents have shown that, from the young person's perspective, relationships with peers and friends are crucial to their health-related behaviours. Peer networks provide opportunities for practising new behaviours and developing the necessary social skills for interactions with same-sex and opposite-sex friends. Adams (1983) pointed out three areas of growth in social competencies that can be gained from peer group participation: first, a growth in social knowledge through learning the appropriate emotional status to adopt in various social contexts; second, a growth in the ability to express empathy with others; third, a growing belief in the power of self-initiation (that is, a state of self-confidence in presenting and carrying out plans within one's group). However, the price for group acceptance is conformity to the peer group in matters such as fashion, dress, personal appearance, musical tastes and leisure activities. Friendships, as Youniss and Smollar (1985) pointed out, are based on completely different sets of structural relationships from those with adults: they are more symmetrical, involving reciprocity, and are evolutionary through adolescence. At the beginning of adolescence there is a move to intimacy in friendships that includes the development of a more exclusive focus, openness to self-disclosure and the sharing of problems and advice. Youniss and Smollar (1985) commented that the central notion is that friends tell one another and get to know just about everything that is going on in one another's lives. Friends literally reason together in order to organise experience and define themselves as persons.

Given the important dynamic developmental role of peer relationships in adolescence it is vital to stress, as have Coggans and McKellar (1994) in a different context, the need to understand the way in which young people select peers, in terms of similar qualities and identities, rather than seeing the peer group as a pressure point which forces young people into particular risky behaviours. This idea of peer preference, to reflect and reaffirm the mid-adolescent's developing ideas of self-identity, can be further extended by our findings.

7 'It's a balance'

Young people speak out about health risk areas in their lives

Introduction

There have been long debates in the academic press about the nature of peer pressure in respect of certain health-risk activities (for example smoking, alcohol use, drug use, sexual activity) and we focus in this chapter on these, not least because it was in the context of these issues that young people themselves spoke most often about the dilemmas and choices with which they were confronted.

Hendry and Kloep (1996) have outlined the importance of socially oriented risk-taking behaviours. It is obvious that very few risk or risky behaviours are carried out alone. They need an audience to be elicited. Thus they are performed in order to demonstrate behaviours to the group so that the individual can secure a place within the group hierarchy. Once that is achieved, it can be less necessary to continue such behaviours. In order to find his or her place in a peer group and to establish a social position the adolescent has to demonstrate certain qualities which are compatible with the group's characteristics and behaviour patterns (Coggans and McKellar, 1994).

While problematic thrill-seeking behaviour may be (because of cultural pressures) more typically a male activity, risk behaviours in order to impress the peer group can be found in both genders. Boys are more likely to try to impress by showing their strength and aggression while girls are more likely to try to be successful with the opposite sex or to be academic achievers. Though the traditional socially motivated stereotypic risk-taking behaviours of boys attract more official attention, girls put themselves at risk to no less a degree.

Linked to these group-focused risk behaviours Hendry and Kloep discussed what they called irresponsible behaviours. By this they meant risk-taking behaviours that are not performed because of the risk they imply, but in spite of it, in order to achieve other goals. Such irresponsible behaviours demonstrate the inability of individuals to see long-term consequences, or, if these are apparent, to be unable to abstain from them because of the short-term 'advantages' perceived to be gained. Examples of these behaviours are smoking and drinking, abstaining from exercise, or engaging in unprotected sex. It is obvious that behaviours such as getting drunk or failing to use condoms are attractive not because of the risk they imply, but for other reasons that temporarily are more important and salient than any possible longer-term negative consequences.

We turn now to look more specifically at young people's beliefs and behaviour patterns on a number of health issues.

Smoking

The Social Survey Division of the Office of Population Censuses and Survey has carried out a series of studies of smoking amongst secondary school children (for example Marsh *et al.*, 1986). A number of problems emerge in looking at this data, not least of which is the fact that 'regular' smoking is defined as smoking at least one cigarette a week, a category threshold so low as to be intuitively rather worrying. From these figures, however, it appears that amongst the adolescent population the prevalence of 'regular' smoking has indeed declined. Goddard (1989) in a study of schoolchildren found that adolescents were much more likely to be smokers if other people at home smoked. Brothers and sisters appeared to have more influence in this respect than did parents. These results are confirmed in a study of Scottish adolescents (Glendinning *et al.*, 1992).

Coggans *et al.* (1991) undertook a large-scale prevalence study as part of a national evaluation of drug education. The young people in this study were all in the second, third or fourth year of their secondary school careers and were identified as representa-

tive of the range both of social class and drug education experience typifying school pupils in these age groups. Something like
15 per cent of the Coggans sample smoked at the 'regular' level
(defined by OPCS as at least one cigarette a week). Such a figure
may seem to reverse the trend of decline in smoking in this age
group, but the rise is likely to be a consequence of differences in
sampling procedure. Davies and Coggans (1991) noted the
strangely bimodal distribution of smoking in the adolescent
population, one sizeable group smoking very infrequently (19 per
cent), and the other group (14 per cent) being frequent smokers.
Trends within this dataset replicate those in the OPCS studies. In
other words, older adolescents are more likely to smoke than
younger ones, males are more likely to smoke than females and
young people from lower socio-economic groups are more likely to
smoke than their counterparts in higher socio-economic groups.

Data collected in 1987 on a 15-year-old cohort by MacIntyre
(1989) confirmed the trends noted above. Just over 12 per cent of
15-year-olds in this regional sample claimed to smoke regularly
(quantities were not defined), but the rate varied from 10 per cent
in middle-class districts to 19 per cent in a principally working-
class area, highlighting the social class differences noted above.
Further evidence on the link with social class comes from the
Young People's Leisure and Lifestyles study (Hendry *et al.*,
1993b), in which 19 per cent of 13–24-year-olds considered
themselves to be smokers. Overall in the data a clear trend with
age is discernible, with the proportion of smokers rising to a peak
in the early twenties and then falling slightly. Of most interest,
however, is the fact that social class differences, when measured
in the traditional way by social class of head of household were
non-significant though the trend was in the same direction noted
in other studies ('non-manual' adolescents providing 11 per cent
of regular smokers, and those from a manual background providing 14 per cent of regular smokers). However, for the oldest
four cohorts it was possible to measure *current* social class rather
than class of origin. In other words, the current socio-economic
position occupied by young people themselves at the time of
the survey was measured (e.g. in full-time education, employed
in semi-skilled occupation). Using this measure, significant
differences do emerge in smoking status between groups of

young people engaged in different types of economic activity. For example, only 11–13 per cent of young people in further education or professional and intermediate categories were 'regular' smokers, compared with 28 per cent of the unemployed.

Of most concern to many health educators is the gender patterning of smoking in adolescence which is beginning to emerge. The 1986 OPCS figures (Marsh *et al.*, 1986) show rates in Scotland being higher and a bigger difference appearing between the rates for boys and girls, with girls being more likely to smoke than boys. Among those who do smoke, however, boys continue across adolescence to be heavier smokers than girls. A study of school pupils aged 14–15 carried out in the 1980s on a non-representative sample, for instance, found that the average daily consumption of girl smokers was six cigarettes, compared with eight cigarettes for boys (Balding, 1986). Diamond and Goddard (1995) report that from age 13 onwards girls are now twice as likely as boys to be regular smokers, with 41 per cent of girls being placed in the regular smoker category as opposed to 23 per cent of boys.

Given this background of statistics what does the evidence from our interviews with adolescents show about both prevalence and attitudes to smoking amongst young people? Those young people who engaged in discussion on the topic of smoking were either strongly 'against' or half-heartedly 'for'. Those against cited yellow skin, bad breath and a range of other 'unlovely' physical symptoms as good reasons for not becoming smokers, but awareness of health risks was high, and the understanding of some of the social circumstances in which a habit might develop quite sophisticated:

> The only reason my mum doesn't smoke is because her mum and dad don't smoke, but you're more likely to smoke if one of your parents smoke . . .   (TA, girl)

This girl and her father are smokers:

> The bad things about smoking are that it can kill you and makes your fingers go yellow, gives you a bad cough and bad breath. The good things are that the taste is nice and some people like doing it because their chums are doing it.
>
>   (ST, girl)

My dad says he can't give me a lecture about it because he was smoking when he was 13. He could give me the points about it but he says he can't give me a lecture about it.   (ST, girl)

Several people used the comparison with smoking 'hash' to illustrate the harmfulness of cigarette smoking in comparison with other forms of behaviour. However, in general from the young person's perspective there was nothing particularly exciting (or forbidden) about smoking cigarettes.

Many young people will experiment with smoking, but with no intention of it developing into a habit.

I've tried smoking because I go around with a girl that smokes. . . . My parents think that if my friends go and smoke, drink or do drugs then I will too.   (JB, girl)

Many of the young people interviewed described themselves to us as non-smokers, but then later declared that they had in fact smoked that week or that they habitually smoked when drunk. These occasions clearly did not count! Their own image of themselves was as non-smokers. Few saw themselves as in any danger of addiction from such casual experimentation or infrequent use, though it was clear that social groupings in leisure settings provided a context for occasional forays into smoking. Again, the interactions among individuals, social and cultural elements are clear.

Alcohol use

The literature on young people drinking describes such behaviour as part of the socialisation process from child to adult (Stacey and Davies, 1970; Barnes, 1977; Sharp and Lowe, 1989). In England and Wales, the majority of adolescents have had their first 'proper' drink by the age of 13 (82 per cent of boys, and 77 per cent of girls). In Scotland, fewer schoolchildren are apparently introduced to alcohol at this age (71 per cent of 12-year-old boys and 57 per cent of girls) but catch up with their English and Welsh peers by the age of 15 (Marsh *et al.,* 1986). Lest these young drinkers cause great concern, it needs to be pointed out that most only drank alcohol a few times a year. More recent data (Goddard, 1996) shows that from age 12 onwards more boys than girls are likely to be drinking at least once a week, and that there is considerable national variation in the patterning, with smaller percentages of Scots young people being involved in regular drinking for example (21 per cent of Scottish boys as opposed to 26 per cent of English boys being regular drinkers), but with this smaller number consuming on average more units of alcohol per week (10.6 units as opposed to 7.4 units for the English boys). The patterning is similar for girls.

Most adolescents' early drinking is done at home with parents. Only as they grow older does the context for their drinking spread to parties, then clubs and discos and lastly to pubs. Scottish adolescents are much less likely than their English and Welsh counterparts to drink in pubs. Marsh *et al.* comment:

> Among the younger Scottish adolescents, particularly the 14- and 15-year-olds, the proportion who claim usually to drink in pubs is small, less than half the values claimed in England and Wales. Scottish adolescents are far more likely to say they drink 'elsewhere'. Since this is not at home, nor on licensed premises, 'elsewhere' must be mostly outside on the streets, or wherever else Scottish adolescents may drink unobserved by parents or authorities.   (1986: 19)

Most young people's drinking is done at weekends, in the company of friends. In relation to quantities, girls in every age group drank less than boys in the OPCS (1986) survey (Marsh *et al.*, 1986). Boys' consumption grows annually, with some very high levels being reached by age 17, whereas girls' consumption peaks in the last year of schooling. In Scotland, boys on average drink three times more than girls.

Data from the Hendry *et al.*'s (1993b) survey confirm the trends noted above, with 5 per cent of 13–14-year-olds being 'frequent drinkers' (once a week or more often), rising to 48 per cent of 17–18-year-olds and 66 per cent of 23–24 year olds (which would obviously include students). In this sample 65 per cent of 17–18-year-olds went to a pub once a month or more. Pub-going seemed to peak in the late teens and thereafter tail off. No significant differences emerged in drinking behaviour over the whole sample in terms of gender although, in the youngest two cohorts, boys were more likely to be frequent drinkers and to be buying alcohol from supermarkets. Across the whole sample there were no significant differences in drinking prevalence by social class of head of household. An analysis of the drinking data for the oldest four cohorts by a residential neighbourhood classification, ACORN (Shaw, 1984) showed raised levels of frequent drinking in the most affluent areas, but this was not statistically significant. Analysis by school catchment of the youngest groups of children did, however, show significant variability. The Highlands and Islands catchments showed the smallest proportion of youngsters who never drank. Two of these three catchments also held the highest proportions of frequent drinkers (approximately 16 per cent of those who drank). The proportion of frequent drinkers ranged between 2 per cent and 18 per cent, indicating the variety of local 'cultures' within which young people drink.

While the long-term health consequences of regularly drinking large amounts of alcohol are well understood, there are also short-term health and social consequences of infrequent but very heavy drinking. Consequently some of the data on 'drunkenness' may actually be of more interest. In the OPCS survey (Marsh *et al.*, 1986) about 30 per cent of the youngest boys and 23 per cent of the youngest girls who drank in Scotland admitted to being 'very drunk' once or more than once. Bearing in mind the caveat that such measurements are very subjective, it would seem that such behaviour peaks for both boys and girls at age 15, but declines more rapidly for girls thereafter.

The introduction of alco-pops has created a new style of drinks aimed at the teenage market and it is perhaps too early to comment on the impact on young people's drinking patterns. The majority of adolescents associate drinking with positive reactions, but Marsh *et al.* (1986) noted that associated with such specific bouts of drunkenness were not only the inevitable physical symptoms but also drinking-related problems such as vandalism, attracting the attention of the police and so on. Coffield (1992) in a more up-to-date study of young people in the northeast of England notes that a pattern of weekend 'binges' appeared to be widespread among both young men and young women and that under-age drinking seemed to be endemic throughout the region. As a result of drinking too much, boys became involved in fights among themselves, with other male groups and with the police; they also damaged themselves and others in accidents with motorbikes and cars; their relationships with parents became strained, and some became more willing to experiment with illicit drugs after drinking heavily. If any of the girls became involved with the police, it was in connection with drink-related offences.

> Among the young people we met, the non-drinker is the deviant and talk of sensible drinking is openly ridiculed. Our young people reported very few hangovers, although they were often sick as a result of excessive drinking. They tend to dismiss any possible health risks because they 'bounce back' so quickly and without any apparent ill-effects.
>
> (Coffield, 1992: 2)

What were the patterns of behaviour and general attitudes to alcohol among the young people we interviewed? The pressure on young people to imitate others in respect of their use of drink or to behave similarly would seem to be fairly strong. As a result young people may occasionally be put in a position of trying to pretend that they are more knowledgeable than they really are when faced with adult questions:

> People talk about some drinks and I don't know what they are but I just go along with the conversation.   (LB, girl)

A recurrent factor in many of the interviews is the wish by young people to be popular. Being popular is often equated with being 'cool' and being cool is synonymous with belonging to youth groups who engage in 'deviant' behaviour, such as drinking, smoking and taking drugs. Amongst boys in particular, the desire to conform, and to be accepted within a group was strong. Frequently as a result of not conforming, individuals were ostracised and isolated on the fringes of their friendship network:

> I could go out and do the drinking and drug-taking scene, which would make me more popular. If you avoid it, it doesn't seem like you are having much fun to the people. There is still a lot of pressure to partake in drink and drugs. I must bore them [friends] sometimes because I'm immature and don't go out

drinking. If you are 15 years old and don't drink, there's not a lot to do. They [his friends] accept it now, they don't look down on me now. (SG, boy)

A lot of pressure to try things out. . . . If you don't get drunk and don't smoke (the drugs thing doesn't matter so much) people laugh at you. You are sad (a sad person) if you don't drink or don't smoke. . . . To be popular you need to smoke, drink and do things you're not supposed to do. The boring people never do any of these things. (CB, boy)

In a way it's good, my girlfriend drinks though she doesn't encourage me. Everyone's doing it. Smoking, drinking and being stoned are perceived as being cool. Being cool is not important to me. My friends see smoking as cool . . . not to be an outcast. It's a balance you have to find yourself. I don't smoke but I drink, it's a balance. (SmG, boy)

I started drinking when I was about 13. Just with friends . . . I wanted to try it. I think it was [because of] my friends [that I started], but I wouldn't let my friends pressure me into taking drugs or that. I think that's worse than drinking.

(LG, girl)

So some pressure is clearly exerted on young people from their friendship group, though they may themselves have made a choice to be part of that particular social network. Social acceptability rests on accepting and participating in some of the rituals that determine group norms. By achieving a 'balance', the adolescent is not faced with the need to be involved in all the activities of the group. Some perceived that there are advantages to acting out 'deviant' behaviours within a group setting in that it can provide 'a safety net':

I enjoy getting drunk as long as I am with my mates as they know when to stop. (BG, boy)

While some young people ostentatiously eschew such behaviours and resist peer pressure (often with a great deal of help and support from their parents) there is often a note of wistfulness in the way they describe the behaviour of others. One boy studying to be a doctor, contemplates the volume of homework that he faces and the restrictions placed on him by his ambition and that of his (Chinese origin) parents for him, and comments:

> It annoys me seeing all these people lazing about drinking and I've got all this homework to do and they are having a great time and I'm not. I suppose later on they'll find the consequences of it.   (SG, boy)

To over-emphasise peer pressure and group norms, however, is to overlook the fact that the majority of young people view alcohol and its use in a very positive way. It 'lubricates' social situations in just the way that a 15-year-old – or any one of us – might need, it can be pleasant in itself, it can be fun to experiment:

> A lot more folk loosen up. They're tense but when they're drunk, they loosen up. You can speak to them better.
> (LiG, girl)

> I enjoy getting drunk. It's like a buzz. It feels like I haven't got a care in the world. It just gets me away from all the hassles with my dad.   (LiG, girl)

> It's like growing up . . . you want to do more things. You want to experiment, like the smoking . . .   (BL, girl)

The sociocultural dilemma of whether or not to drink alcohol was clearly much more important in young people's perceptions than issues about sexual behaviour or drugs. Almost all groups discussed the role of parents in initiating or modelling 'appropriate' drinking behaviour. For most, this meant parents allowing them occasional drinks (usually of relatively low alcohol content) on social or family occasions, with the view that this would help them to learn how to handle a social drug sensibly:

> I only do it when my mum and dad is around because they know I'm doing it and they let me do it.   (TG, girl)

> Boy A: My dad usually gives me a can of beer when we are watching the football, just as long as he is there.
>
> Boy B: My dad encourages me sometimes. He says it's a good idea to get it in young, 'cos when you're 18, you'll just get drunk all the time.

Many parents appeared to bargain with their offspring, as we discuss in a different chapter, allowing them the indulgence of misusing alcohol on the understanding that if they got their 'kicks' this way they might be less likely to experiment with drugs. Alcohol is thus interpreted as a normal or acceptable drug whose impact is understood, as opposed to newer forms of drugs, the impact of which (in the long term or the short term) is not easily understood by parents or young people. People clearly feel they can 'control' alcohol use, whereas drugs create a fear that their use may not be controllable or predictable.

In some circumstances parents demonstrated through their own behaviour how to handle hangovers or the consequences of over-indulgence:

> Take a drink of water to get the body balance back up. That's what my mum does [giggles]. That's how I know.
>
> (TA, girl)

Only one or two of the youngsters we spoke to admitted that they had actually drunk to excess themselves. Many were scathing about people who got themselves into a state where they 'lost control' and where they couldn't later remember what they'd done or said:

> I don't like it when I hear my older friends who are coming home saying they're feeling rough. It's cool to say 'I'm feeling rough'. . . . You're just making a fool of yourself. I haven't been drunk very often but you do say things you regret. You're scared to see your friends the next day.   (AA, girl)

There were clearly major differences, however, in local cultures of drinking, which combine with both personal and group prefer-ences to create a complex picture of drinking patterns in mid-adolescence.

Drug misuse

One of the forms of drug misuse associated with younger adoles-cents is solvent misuse. Misuse of solvents is discouraged both because of the short-term and long-term dangers to health and safety that they present. One of the characteristic features of solvent misuse is that it is often very localised and very transitory, becoming wildly popular with a cohort of young people on a particular estate or in a school, for instance, then quickly disappearing. So, in some places at some times, large numbers of children will be experimenting, but only a few of these young people will carry on misusing solvents after the 'fad' has passed. British studies (Ives, 1990a) suggest that between 4 per cent and 8 per cent of secondary school pupils have tried solvents, and that sniffing peaks around ages 13–15. In Davies and Coggans' sample, nearly 11 per cent of the sample had used solvents at least once although less than 1 per cent reported using solvents once a month or more frequently. Most of those who had used solvents had used them only once or a few times (Davies and Coggans, 1991).

However, despite the low incidence of continued misuse, it is clear that the fashion for solvent misuse has not gone away despite attracting less media attention in recent years. Numbers of solvent-related deaths give some indication of the problem's continuation. In 1983, when concern was at its highest, deaths totalled eighty-two. In 1988 there were 134 deaths, more deaths per annum than are attributed to the misuse of any other illegal drug in the adolescent population (Wright, 1991). Part of the concern rests in the fact that published guidelines to retailers on the sale of glues – the most well-known solvent – have led to a trend towards misuse of more dangerous products such as aerosols (Ives, 1990b; Ramsey, 1990).

More common in usage among adolescents is cannabis, ranking third behind alcohol and cigarettes as a preferred drug. Davies and Coggans (1991) note that although 15 per cent of their sample of school-age children had tried cannabis at least once, only 2 per cent carried on using it about once a month or more frequently.

Cannabis is not in itself addictive and, although linked with short-term memory problems and other minor symptoms, is not associated with any significant long-term damage to health. It is, however, an illegal substance, and thus most of the problems associated with its use stem from social rather than medical causes. There is some evidence that young people view cannabis in quite a different light from those offering health education on the topic (Hendry *et al.*, 1991). Those concerned with health promotion for young people are often bound by professional guidelines to group cannabis with other illegal drugs and must effectively prohibit its use. Young people's own culture, however, denies that cannabis is harmful – it is often seen as less dangerous than alcohol, both in terms of the quantities consumed and the fact that it is less likely than alcohol to provoke violent behaviour. The association of cannabis with other illegal substances diminishes the validity of the message that health educators promote. The study reported by Davies and Coggans (1991) demonstrates how low is the incidence of other illegal drugs in school-age populations. Six per cent reported having used LSD at least once. Figures for heroin and cocaine were 1 per cent. Ecstasy was recorded at below 1 per cent of young people having used it, although more recent surveys might highlight the fashion of use of such designer drugs in dance settings. Amphetamines or 'speed' have, however, replaced 'E' as a popular choice with young people, at least in one area in Scotland (Fast Forward, 1994a), or 'E' is used in combination with other drugs to 'bring young people down' after an all-night rave.

Our discussions with young people around these topics generally revealed a huge level of ignorance and a lack of awareness of the characteristics of drugs. A group of boys in a residential school was the only exception to this rule. Characteristically groups spoke about 'drugs' in general, rather than naming specific types of drugs and their effects, for instance, and the only drug to receive any substantial attention and which they talked about among themselves was 'hash'. Clearly few of them had personally tried anything else. Many seemed blithely unaware of the networks for dealing or the extent to which parents and press felt they were exposed to the 'drugs menace'. There were clear differences in the extent to which drugs were seen to be available and being used within different areas, with middle-class, suburban and rural areas still far less exposed than inner-city areas:

Girl A: Half of my chums have tried all sorts of drugs. I haven't tried nothing.

Girl B: Most of my chums have tried a lot of drugs as well but I just could nae touch it.

Even on the subject of cannabis, which did exercise them, there was doubt as to whether this made one more or less aggressive, whether it was more or less addictive than ordinary cigarette tobacco, and so on. They were not expert, though they were not resistant to experimenting with friends. It was clearly not perceived as particularly dangerous:

> Hash is more acceptable than smoking because smoking damages your health so much. People say hash doesn't kill you or damage your health. I don't really believe that. I don't think either are sensible.   (AA, girl)

KT, girl: I've tried hash. It just relaxes you.

ST, girl: They say hash is worse than cigarettes. You get more addicted.

KT, girl: I dinna ken.

ST, girl: You read in the newspapers every day people aged nine or ten on hash already. I mean it's terrible. I mean, I know so is smoking. But you can get more addicted to hash than to cigarettes. You can get killed by taking drugs or hash more than you can by smoking a cigarette.

The whole issue is very complex:

> Heaps of folk drink and do drugs. I don't like drink much. I've had drugs, speed and hash and I smoke ten fags a day. My mates tried to get me to drink but I didn't like the taste. Drugs are all right. It's usually at discos. I take speed to keep awake. I just buy off friends what I need for the day. I wouldn't try cocaine or stuff like that. I tried half an 'E', not really into that. I hate tabs, they make me freak out. I took half a tab once and the walls came alive. I started 'cos my mates took them as well. The last time I took speed it put me off a bit 'cos I was up the next day and couldn't eat or nothing. I think my Dad suspects. It's the risk that's good with drugs. I wouldn't want to be caught and charged.   (SC, boy)

Few mentioned pressure from peers to take 'hash', although

drug-taking was clearly perceived to be associated with certain groups or 'types' of young people or types of lifestyle:

There are particular groups into drugs . . . the 'heavies' and the 'casuals', although the latter are only into it on a Friday night and it's not as much as it used to be.   (AA, girl)

A lot of people drink, smoke and get drunk. Quite a few take drugs but not dangerous drugs. They get drunk a lot of the time. A lot of people smoke, a lot of people whose parents think they're perfect smoke at school. I've not tried any except alcohol. I never get drunk though. There is a lot of pressure to try things out, if you don't get drunk and don't smoke, people laugh at you. You are sad if you don't get drunk or don't smoke. I don't believe in it though. Only one of my friends drinks and smokes. She wants to be popular. Her sister puts a lot of pressure on her to do these things. To be popular you need to smoke, drink and do things you're not supposed to do. The boring people never do any of these things.   (CD, girl)

It is often claimed that young people who go to raves, take 'E'. Yet, in this conversation this assumption is challenged:

LyG, girl: Everyone thinks that if you go to raves you take drugs. But you go to raves and you don't take drugs.

LiG, girl: Everybody says I won't be able to dance for the full time so I'll just take some speed and that'll get me going. I turn round and say well I can manage it and I think you can too. Me and some of my pals can manage to dance all night in that hall. All night without stopping, without taking drugs or alcohol. For them it's an excuse to take something.

It would appear that cultural 'shifts' towards the 'normalisation' of drug-usage has filtered down to the young, and this combines with certain group settings which reinforce the adolescents' desire to experiment with activities seen as symbolically 'adult'.

Sexual activity

Adolescent sexual behaviour has always been a cause of concern to adults in society. Fears about sexual activity leading to unwanted pregnancy are coupled with a desire to protect younger adolescents from exploitation and pressure to become sexually active before they have the emotional or social maturity to cope. Apart from risks to mental and social well-being, there are risks to health both in the short term and the long term. Early pregnancies are associated with increased risk for both mother and baby; early onset of sexual behaviour has been statistically linked in females with cancers of the reproductive organs appearing in later life, and sexually transmitted diseases pose threats to the health and well-being of young people of both sexes. In recent years, of course, the spread of HIV through sexual activity has caused an increased focus to be placed on young people's social activities. Bury (1991: 43) comments that teenagers are often regarded as key factors in the future of the heterosexual epidemic because of myths about their sexual behaviour, as they are often seen as promiscuous and irresponsible in their attitude to protection.

The assumption that young people do consider themselves invulnerable has become a popular, if not a standard, part of current beliefs about youth, typified in work such as that of Elkind (1984), who developed the idea of the 'Personal Fable'. Elkind suggested that the Personal Fable can be positive and productive as well as potentially damaging. This is because it may, in Plant and Plant's words, 'inspire adolescents to aim for exceptional goals, which some in fact do manage to attain' (1992: 114). They acknowledge, however, that on the negative side, it may also encourage young people to ignore reasonable precautions, like the use of contraception.

The difficulties in obtaining accurate information either on sexual behaviours or on HIV status are too well known to need rehearsing. There have been two major studies of young people's sexual behaviour in Britain, one in the mid-1960s (Schofield, 1965) and the other ten years later (Farrell, 1978). Since then most other studies have been localised and small-scale, apart from Johnson *et al.*'s (1994) research which included questions concerning age of first intercourse, sexual experience and lifestyles.

Earlier Ford (1987) identified the important indicators of patterns of heterosexual activity as age at first intercourse, the level of pre-marital sex, the number of sex partners and the proportion using a condom. With regard to the first of these, the trend has been for teenagers to begin sexual intercourse at a younger age than in the past (for example Farrell, 1978; Ford and Bowie, 1989). Johnson *et al.* (1994) have shown that the age for first heterosexual intercourse reveals a pattern of decreasing age at occurrence, together with an increase in the proportions reporting sexual experience before the age of 16, together with some convergence in the behaviour of young men and young women over time. In the past four decades the median age at first heterosexual intercourse has fallen from 21 to 17 years for women and from 20 to 17 years for men, while the proportion reporting its occurrence before the age of 16 has increased from fewer than 1 in a hundred of women now aged 55 years and over, to nearly one in five of those now in their teens.

Social class differences in early sexual experience were significant in the 1970s, with young working-class men significantly more likely than their middle-class counterparts to be sexually experienced, but these differences appear to be less significant in more recent data collections (MORI, 1990; Wellings and Bradshaw, 1994; Wight, 1993). These changes need to be seen in the context of liberalising legal reforms, advances in medical technology and changes in a permissive direction of social and sexual attitudes. The general impression seems to be one of increasing homogeneity with respect to gender, occupational and educational levels and other socio-demographic variables. Early intercourse is still associated with lower social class and low educational levels, but these effects are weakening. This is also true of 'current' social class (i.e. based on the young person's current level of economic activity rather than 'ascribed' social class (i.e. based on the occupation of the father). Ford and Bowie's (1989) work, for instance, suggests that those in full-time education are twice as likely not to have had sexual intercourse as those in full-time employment, housewives or the unemployed.

It is important to stress the vast diversity in the individual experiences of young people. Conger and Petersen (1984) make a particular point of emphasising the importance of looking at individual differences when considering figures such as these. Apart from age, gender, socio-economic status and nationality, variables such as social class, ethnic origin and cultural background will obviously play their part in determining sexual behaviour. The broad social trends described above also need to be considered in the light of other studies which have highlighted the different experience of young people in urban and rural settings (Johnson *et al.*, 1994). Ford and Bowie (1989) found only 56 per cent of youngsters in rural areas were sexually experienced compared with 70 per cent of their counterparts in urban and semi-urban areas.

Although teenagers are more likely to be sexually experienced than they have been in the past, there is no evidence that they are more likely to have casual sex relationships. Ford and Morgan (1989) claim that over 70 per cent of teenagers have intercourse only within a committed, loyal relationship. Bury (1984) and Wellings and Bradshaw (1994) have characterised adolescent sexual relationships as being 'serial monogamy'. Other studies seem to confirm this pattern (Abrams *et al.*, 1990). Such a claim would seem to be borne out by Stegen's (1983) and Tobin's (1985) studies of female teenage family planning clinic attendees. This evidence, now ten years old, showed that approximately 90 per cent of those attending had only one or two sexual partners, and they were clearly 'comfortable' with the social acceptance of their sexual activity.

Johnson *et al.* (1994) also report that first intercourse is now often associated with more planning and less spontaneity than formerly. They state that the majority of young people have their first experience of sexual intercourse within an established relationship. Young women are usually initiated by an older male partner, while young men's first partners tend to be age peers. It is uncommon, and increasingly so, for first intercourse to take place within marriage, and very rare for young men's first sexual intercourse to be with a prostitute.

Nevertheless, a small proportion of young people have multiple sexual partners, and it has been claimed that it is a behaviour possibly associated with emotional deprivation or serious psychological problems (Hein *et al.*, 1978). Studies which have focused on 'sexually delinquent' youth (those who have committed sexual offences against other persons) and runaways emphasise the very high-risk pattern of sexual activity common in some groups which requires very targeted and specific health education interventions (Rotherham-Borus *et al.*, 1991). Again there is a boundary problem here as to how significant a problem this is seen to be. MORI (1990) reports that 11 per cent of 16–19-year-olds had four or more sexual partners in the previous year. Although some of these sexual encounters may have been monogamous and not undertaken in a promiscuous fashion at the time, the impact of such activities in increasing the risk factor for young people should be noted by health professionals working with adolescents.

Contraceptive use among teenagers has risen in line with the increase in those claiming sexual experience in teenage years, but such use has been shown in numerous studies to be inconsistent. The condom is the only contraceptive which assists in the prevention of sexually transmitted diseases and the HIV virus. Ford and Bowie (1989) suggest that about a third of sexually active young people use condoms, but almost all claim to use them for contraceptive rather than disease-prevention purposes (Hendry *et al.*, 1991). Despite the campaigning for condom use, a complex web of cultural and social factors conspire to make them unappealing and unusable for many young people, especially when other forms of contraception (for example the pill) are available (Wight, 1990). Despite the fact that contraception is difficult for many young people to access or negotiate with a partner, the evidence of data relating to teenage pregnancies attests to the fact that young women are no more likely now than in the past to conceive children at this early stage in their lives (Johnson *et al.*, 1994).

All of the foregoing relates to heterosexual activity. Very little is known about rates of homosexual activity among adolescents. Kent-Baguley (1990: 106) notes that 'not surprisingly, the majority of young lesbians and gays feel marginalised, isolated and unhappy at school, often feeling obliged to participate in "queerbashing" talk to avoid self-revelation'. Little wonder that the extent of the phenomenon is so unclear. A MORI poll carried out for the Health Education Authority (MORI, 1990) asked 16–19-year-old respondents to place themselves on a scale indicating their sexual orientation. MORI concluded that 88 per cent in this age group were clearly heterosexual and only 1 per cent clearly homosexual. A further 6 per cent, however, were bisexual or had a bisexual orientation. Also in question is the extent to which homosexual practices place young people at risk. Blanket assumptions about the nature of sexual acts or the levels of promiscuity in this subgroup too often reflect simple stereotypes and prejudices. Young people themselves are particularly confused about the nature of the AIDS danger in relation to homosexuality since there is almost no discussion within health education about sexuality *per se* and homosexuality in particular.

What evidence do we have from our own discussions with adolescents about young people's levels of sexual activity or their feelings towards it? Our evidence underlines the need to disaggregate national data and look at local variations. Despite the aggregate national statistics on the number of sexually active young people under the age of 16 (which would imply approximately a third of young people of this age might be sexually active), our investigations found few young people admitting to being engaged in sexual activity except in working-class urban catchment areas. There seemed to be a consensual feeling that though there might be a lot of talk, there was not a lot of action amongst young people of this age! Indeed there were strong views expressed by girls about the inappropriateness (as well as the illegality) of sexual activity for 15-year-olds:

Girl A: I wouldn't be doing it at my age because I'm still far too young. What is the age?

Girl B: I don't think it should be 16. It's far too young. I think it should be 21 to have sex for the first time because that's when most people have matured a lot more. At 16 they're still practically babies.

The prevailing attitude was that the girls either thought themselves too young for sex or that it was not worth the risk before they were 16. EA discusses sex with her mum:

We talk about sex all the time. She's always saying 'If you ever come to me and say you are pregnant, I'm going to be really annoyed.' I say, 'But Mum, sex is something that comes with university.' She says, 'Well, I'm glad you feel like that. You're only 14, you've got a long way to go, you've got a lot of living to do before you make decisions like that.'

Most striking is the disparity in maturity between girls and boys from the same age cohort. One suspects that the boys, looking for younger partners themselves, were less involved in the dating and mating game than girls of a comparable chronological age.

Girls clearly discuss sexual matters among themselves, but they are very careful about their reputations. Almost no one spoke about pressure to have sex being exerted either by female peers or by older boyfriends, except that the girls' group in one rural area identified girls with a certain lifestyle (the 'casuals') as being most likely to be pressured into sex as part of the way of proving their status within the style group.

There was little or no evidence of promiscuous behaviour or intent. Virtually all girls were explicit about not wishing to become sexually involved with boys on a casual basis. In one catchment only was there much talk of other people they knew having sex. LG believed there were a lot of people having sex in her year, and it was suspected that one girl in her class was pregnant.

The boys' perception of relationships was quite different. They perceived that girls were under pressure to have sex. For their own part it was clear that the subject of sex was one which troubled them greatly. In contrast to the girls' certainty about their attitude and their locus of control, boys clearly felt threatened by peer pressure not to reveal their virgin status, or to actually go out and 'prove themselves' in some way. There was much more talk about 'saving face'.

If you don't lie everyone would rip the piss out of you.

(CB, boy)

One feels also that boys are essentially isolated at this stage. Unable to talk to each other about their anxieties for fear of making revelations about themselves they talk wistfully of the girls being 'more together' on such matters:

Boy A: Girls spend more time talking about it than boys.
Boy B: Boys get embarrassed when they talk about that; girls dinna.

Pregnancy could not be further from their minds at this stage. The boys' reaction to the thought that they or someone they knew well might have fathered a child was stark fear. They would run! There was much talk among boys and girls of home pregnancy kits – these are obviously a source of some curiosity and mystique, but, reassuringly perhaps, there was also mention from both boys and girls of the need to seek out an adult mentor should this predicament arise.

The isolation of the boys was keenly illustrated in considering who they might talk to about the process of puberty. The idea that any such discussion might take place among 'mates' was soundly rejected. It was even felt that parents would make a fool of you were you to ask questions of them. Other studies have implied that girls and women often become the principal sources of information and education for boys and men on health issues. Clearly the boys' isolation and need for knowledge is not served well by the health education methods in common use in schools. Boys revealed to us that much of the input on sexual matters, for instance, had been both premature and even frightening:

Boy A: We were shown a woman's body cells dividing in first year. It's all complicated . . . like the cells. . . . It's not like how to get stuck in.

Boy B: We got a video in first year. There was a woman naked. The camera went right inside her. It wasn't very nice at first year at that age.

Now, at the age of 15, it still didn't answer their need to know more about the mechanics and the necessary relational skills rather than the values, and it was also clear that they felt that too much overt interest on their part in the form of asking questions might be seen as revealing an eagerness or engagement with the topic which would be viewed as highly suspicious:

If it is a really serious thing like sex you would nae like to ask your parents because they would then automatically think that you had done it and then they would start saying, 'No, I don't want you doing any of this.'   (AA, boy)

One of the major features for us appeared to be the lack of information that boys have and their inability to obtain information. Often there is a ritual where direct questions are taboo and only covert methods of inquiry are acceptable, for fear of 'losing face' or being rebuked by friends. Young men were asked how they acquired information about sex:

> My mates. I'd drop hints and they'd fill in the rest. . . .
>
> (BG, boy)

> Girls are far more informed than boys are. It's because of the magazines, definitely. Boys are far more likely to believe all the rubbish that is going around the playground.　　(KA, girl)

> I can talk to my best friend about it but my other friends laugh at you. All my teachers are dead old so I wouldn't talk to them. I might talk to a girl but I'd have to be drunk.　　(ShG, boy)

> There's things you want to know but can't find out. My mum and dad gave me a book on the birds and the bees.
>
> (ShG, boy)

> I always carry a condom in my pocket but I've never been asked to. I am worried about sex in general. I don't feel confident, like my friends, one of them has done it and he never says anything about it. He just said 'it was over dead fast' but never said like what you do. If I really wanted to find out I'd go to the FPA or doctors but I wouldn't go there 'cos it's embarrassing 'cos you're too young and my mum doesn't expect me to do it.　　(ShG, boy)

Most young people were glaringly ignorant about sexually transmitted diseases. The only one most of them could name was HIV/AIDS:

> I've no knowledge, whatsoever, apart from obtaining them from sex. I'd ask my friends. If they didn't know, I'd ask my sister.　　(CB, boy)

On the face of it, AIDS is not a big issue for these young people. Reasons include lack of sexual activity, trusting a group, not knowing anyone who has it.

> Doesn't affect me as I'm not having sex with anyone. As long as you are careful.　　(GB, boy)

I'm not bothered about it. I don't know anyone who's got it.

(AK, boy)

You see it [AIDS] on the TV and in the papers but you think it will never happen to me. If you are going to have sex with someone you don't stop and think, what if I catch AIDS off you. That's a total downer on it.   (GG, girl)

AIDS worries me but if I was drunk it wouldn't bother me.

(ShG, boy)

'Cos I mean, it doesn't really bother me. If anyone has got it, you can't get it if you kiss someone. I know how you get it. I'm not exactly going to be having sex the age I am. I mean even if I knew someone who had AIDS, I would stick by them and wouldn't leave them.   (ST, girl)

As long as you take the right precautions, the chance is you won't get it. It's something you can stop.   (RG, girl)

I don't talk to my friends about AIDS. We don't think anyone of us has got AIDS. You would never think a 15-year-old girl and a 17-year-old boy would have AIDS in Banchory. You don't think it will happen to you. No one has slept with anyone outside the group so it would be contained within the group.   (SB, girl)

While AIDS did not seem a big concern, when the young people were questioned closely there was some recognition of worry and personal concern:

I do sometimes think about AIDS or cancer if we're watching a programme about it and I think about it afterwards. It's worrying.   (MA, girl)

The only thing I worry about at the moment is AIDS in case my friends get it. Though they're not having sex or anything, just if they ever went into hospital and got it through a blood transfusion. I would stick by them but I would worry how other people would treat them.   (EA, girl)

Aye, I worry, I don't want to catch it. It's passed on through infected blood and saliva. It's not covered in social education classes.   (RK, boy)

One girl who admitted having sex when drunk was vowing never to drink again. She had been scared not at the thought of getting pregnant but because, when she told her mother that she had had sex, her mother had been frightened by the prospect of AIDS. While the girl knew about AIDS, in fact she said she had given her mum all the facts about it, she admitted it had not crossed her mind that she might have been infected until her mum brought it up. While she is aware that the prevailing advice is to use a condom, she thinks the advice is unrealistic:

> Everyone says use a condom. You've not got time to think about it. If you're like K, if you want it, you have it. The thing is I didn't want it but I didn't want to say no. We just got on with it. They don't ask you 'Would you like to have sex tonight? I'll use a condom for you.' It would just put you off.

In such settings young people do not think clearly (nor do adults!) and there is a need for social skills and assertiveness training to assist them with problematic situations.

Attitudes to homosexuality were mixed, with girls, on the whole, expressing more understanding:

ST, girl:	If someone is homosexual, you should give them a chance, you shouldn't say 'I'm not talking to you because you're gay.' Shouldn't do things like that. You should give them a chance to prove otherwise.
QUESTIONER:	To prove what?
ST, girl:	To prove that they can handle themselves. To prove that they won't try anything. Because some people won't go near gay people in case they try anything.

Boys, according to ST, make fun of homosexuality. 'But you just ignore them.' This is borne out in another school where they have discussions in Religious Education.

> I don't know if the boys believe what they say that all gays should be hung up. Maybe they just say it to make them sound macho. There is a couple of boys who stand up against the other boys and say I don't think that is right but they have to be really brave to do that. (KB, girl)

She explains further:

> I think it's partly boys thinking they have to. Being called a poof is an insult. I think it's easier for girls to stand up and say what they think against other girls.

Both boys and girls clearly perceived the homophobia of young adolescent males, and their need to voice conformity to heterosexual values. Girls appeared to be more tolerant of variations in gender roles, whereas boys expressed traditional stereotypically sexist views. Such attitudes may stem from the rather isolated socialisation procedures of young men which may encourage male posturing rather than the expression of true feeling.

Concluding comments

Brannen *et al.* (1994) pointed out that young people are one of the healthiest social groups as judged by indicators such as mortality and hospitalisation rates, although their distinctive health problems such as accidents, suicide, external violence and risks attached to teenage pregnancy do give cause for concern. Brannen *et al.* concluded that the main rationale for the plethora of health education interventions targeted at young people do not derive from these statistics but rather from the clustering of health-risk behaviours observed to occur with increasing frequency in the teenage years. Smoking, alcohol consumption, drug taking and unprotected sexual activity are all singled out by adult health educators as topics of particular concern. Petosa (1989) challenged the view of adolescence as a period of development fraught with problems that need to be prevented. He argued that problem-oriented health education often fails to serve the needs of young people, thus compromising programme effectiveness. Instead he suggested a wellness approach with concepts that are defined in terms of, and applied to, the real needs of adolescents. Petosa suggested several indications of wellness. These are: adolescents actively experimenting and stretching their self-concepts in new directions, developing social coping skills to deal with their environments, expanding social competence and friendships, and meaningfully integrating and acknowledging their emerging sexuality as part of their identity.

He concluded that strong peer interaction is an important and healthy part of adolescence. The majority of behaviours supported by peer groups are pro-social and health-enhancing. From a wellness perspective, the understanding of adolescents' behaviour requires an examination of how their actions are meeting their developmental needs. Armed with such understanding Petosa encourages health educators to facilitate changes in adolescent personal and social factors with the aim of ensuring supportive and yet challenging environments.

8 Conclusions
'I'm not going to do anything stupid!'

Introduction

In this final chapter we want to review what young people have told us, by outlining a number of broad themes which emerged from our discussions with mid-adolescents and by considering and interpreting those themes a little more deeply. We conclude the chapter and the book by reviewing why it is critical for young people to be given a voice and why this poses challenges for many who work with young people on a range of issues including health. Can we listen to young people and believe them when they tell us that they won't do anything stupid . . .?

Young people's perceptions of their health needs

First, and most obviously, health is not seen by young people as a major life concern in the same way as adults perceive their health status. Adults' personal concerns relate to feelings of general well-being and the maintenance of good health and are influenced by various sociocultural influences across the life course (Backett and Davison, 1992). Young people's concerns tend to be short-term and to relate to the 'here-and-now'. Therefore young people's perceptions are centred, for example, on their personal and physical appearance, diet and the maintenance of a slim physique, decisions around drinking, smoking and drug use. When we look at issues with regard to sexual relationships and practices and risk-taking, these also figured significantly in young people's discussions with us.

Many of these perceived concerns of mid-adolescence are apparently reflections of wider cultural images. Desirable stereo-types and ideal body types produced in the mass media and the fashion and film scenes are filtered through magazines via glamour and/or pop culture role models, and these impinge on young people. These concerns are reinforced by peer pressures around pop and fashion sub-cultures. The impact of this on young people, despite their general current good state of health, results in 'distorted' views of their physique and appearance and also produces unrealistic ideas about the function of diet and exercise in relation to health, fitness and good appearance. Crash diets and sudden bouts of exercising are the manifestations of their attempts to approximate to these desirable cultural images. Hence there may be some value in considering health behaviours within a broader view of lifestyle development. Young people are either not knowledgeable about good diet and exercise practices or else wilfully ignore them. Cultural images set the scene for poor dieting and exercise behaviours. The possible danger here, expressed in recent media stories, is that such practices may be linked to hunger suppression by the use of drugs, bouts of high activity levels in dancing and at raves, or 'binge' syndromes linked to anorexia or bulimia. Health educators too, in confusing leanness with fitness or wellness, are perhaps guilty of perpetuating these broad influences on young people's attitude to eating.

Community factors

The strong association between different styles of leisure pursuits and young people's health practices was notable in a number of the contexts in which this study was carried out. In some urban settings, the freedom given to young people to wander in a variety of built environments and contexts creates settings allowing experimentation with various types of unhealthy practices without parental checks and balances being readily available. In suburban and rural areas leisure activities were more carefully monitored by parents, with young people 'steered' more towards adult-run clubs and organisations or being driven by parents to sports and community facilities. Such freedom on the one hand,

and constraining factors on the other, creates considerable difference in the lifestyle patterns, in attitudes to health and in health practices of different types of young people.

The patterns of community based leisure pursuits mentioned to us by young people reflected embedded social class values and the different transitional pathways for those mid-adolescents who intended to progress to higher education or who attempted to join early the 'world of work', and projected a life-view of early marriage and family responsibilities. Thus, for the latter (mainly urban working-class) group, early relational and sexual encounters were seen as necessary preliminaries to being able to merge into the local subcultural scene as an adult. Equally, their involvement with smoking and drinking was consistent with the values and norms of the adult communities in which they were growing up.

Parental influences

With regard to parental influences on health, these were perceived to be multi-faceted in that parents could be perceived as positive role models, that is, young people were impressed by parental health practices and copied these and integrated them into their own developing lifestyles. Alternatively, parents could be perceived as negative role models, that is, young people were repelled by parental behaviours and quite deliberately chose alternative behaviour patterns. Finally, parents were often perceived by young people as selective advice givers, that is, parental views on major health issues were not necessarily seen as particular issues for the adolescent.

These patterns of parental influence on health behaviours are further complicated by the fact that parental advice on health is both gendered and structured by social class. Put crudely, and generally, middle-class parents seem to use affection as an emotional bait, giving clear indications that certain behaviours were not approved of. Further, they encouraged deferred gratification in health behaviours, reflecting embedded social class values. Working-class parents on the other hand appeared often to veto young people's actions and behaviour by fairly aggressive and confrontational strategies. Their attempts at harm minimisation

were conducted by focusing on key aspects of their own perceived major health risks.

On the other hand, the approach of working-class parents
might be seen as being more *realistic* in enabling socialisation
into the accepted adult cultural practices of such communities by
teaching young people *over time* to acquire the necessary social
skills in drinking and smoking 'sensibly'.

Peers and friends

Coleman and Hendry (1990) have stressed the important need in
mid-adolescence for peer acceptance, and comments about peer
pressure were particularly noticeable in young people's attitudes
and behaviours as expressed to us. But 'peer pressure' was also
used to explain inappropriate, unhealthy activities. So in a sense
the wider peer network within which young people spend their
day-to-day existence can act as a 'health hazard' in creating
unfavourable norms by both providing incorrect, or indeed false
information and by producing inaccurate expectations about
behaviour at this particular stage of adolescence. However, it was
clear from their comments that many young people do go
through an experimental stage, perhaps in response to peer
expectations and pressure, which passes as they mature and
become more confident in their independence and self-agency.
Such expectations and pressures can create a period of
uncertainty and 'risk' for young people, before they develop the
social skills, self-knowledge and self-competence to withstand (to
some extent) group norms, to pass through group 'initiation'
stages, to find an accepted place in the peer network, and to
develop a realistic knowledge about the behaviours and claims of
others.

By contrast closer friendship groups appeared to develop by
choice and by preference of characteristics and collaborative
activities, and in a sense allowed the young person a reaffirm-
ation of chosen identity in mid-adolescence. They further
enabled young people to perceive, understand and accept the
values of their chosen groupings. This in turn allowed them to be
fairly critical, and even scathing, of the fashion styles, health
behaviours, and general social conduct of other groups. Here was

clear evidence in 'in-group'/'out-group' perceptions which further strengthened and affirmed lifestyle and identity choices. Social reinforcement around a clustering of behaviours and attitudes allowed greater cohesion and selection of friends by preference and by commonalties of hobby interests, dress, leisure interests, attitudes to school, pop music, allegiances, and so on.

Gender and friendships

With regard to friendship, boys and girls in mid-adolescence relate to their companions within group settings in different ways. Girls appear to 'use' friends to develop social skills, rehearse social encounters, share feelings and give advice about social strategies and problems, whereas boys used the group for the sharing of experiences and activities, and to gain social status and reputation. For boys, little is exchanged among group members in terms of information or the sharing of feelings. Rather there is a great deal of exaggerated boasting, particularly in relation to sex, in order to gain group status and a position in the hierarchy. Indeed, our interviews showed that boys would not discuss intimate issues with other boys, but very often would go to discuss their more serious personal concerns with girls with whom they were friendly. With their friends girls show more tolerance to other groups and to other viewpoints than their own in relation to behaviour and health. Boys are fairly intolerant, and need, in a sense, to use this prejudice to prove their conformity and 'traditional' macho conventionality. This became abundantly clear in their attitudes towards homosexuality where in the main they were extremely homophobic.

Information on health matters

Since the sharing of information and feelings differed between friendship groups according to gender, another aspect of our interviewing showed that sources of information differed between the sexes. Girls were much more likely to gain accurate information from a vast array of teenage girls' and women's magazines. Boys tended to rely on pornography and on a 'word of mouth' peer system which on occasions led to an absorption of inaccurate information and the development of sexist stereotypes. The dangers inherent in such exchanges of misinformation are that exaggerated boasting and similar social 'messages' are used as strategies for gaining social status and 'saving face' amongst young men. These exchanges are also often accompanied by externalised aggressive behaviour, which can be a successful short-term strategy in peer group exchanges and it is thus reinforced, thereby encouraging similar strategies to be adopted in future social encounters. A 'double standard' social norm emerges in the sense that 'boasting' girls are seen by peers to violate norms of sexuality and gender. Misinformation often begins from the use of basic sexist stereotypes emerging from pornographic magazines, books and videos which boys often access in the absence of other more reliable local sources of information.

Both genders, however, were united in their views about schools as sources of information in health matters. School materials and the health curriculum and the ways that teachers presented health topics were considered to be inappropriate to their needs. A number of changes in the status of the subject and its presentation would seem to be a very necessary consideration for the future. Young people wanted more up-to-date information, more up-to-date videos and teaching materials and the opportunity to discuss realistically and relevantly the matters that concern them, rather than being given 'information' in a way which does not allow them to discuss in any great detail intimate matters. Schools are important given that they are the only social institution (beyond the family) that almost all young people pass though on their way to adulthood, but it seems to us that it is necessary to carry out a re-examination of the aims, objectives, procedures, processes and professional servicing of school-based health education. In this more attention should be given to young people's views – their need for discussion; their wishes regarding single-sex groupings; and their demands for accurate non-judgemental information, to be allowed to reach their own conclusions on issues, and to learn knowledge and skills appropriate and relevant to their day-to-day lives. The teachers' role in this process also begs consideration, with perhaps a greater need being expressed for teaching–learning collaborations to involve teachers, parents and pupils working together with a range of health and medical professionals from the local community.

Risks and challenges

When we examine the relationship between the influence of the peer group and self-agency of the young, we come to consider a number of aspects related to decision-making in the health sphere. As we mentioned earlier, experimentation in various domains is characteristic of mid-adolescence but what emerges in terms of self-agency is the idea of 'rites of passage'. Young people seem by and large to learn from what on the surface may appear to be an unhappy or negative experience. In resolving not to repeat such an experience in the same manner, they nevertheless gain a reputation within the peer group for having undertaken the actual process of resolving a crisis. Rutter and Smith (1995) have talked about such experiences as 'steeling' activities which enable resilience and the development of coping mechanisms for future use to develop in adolescence. This ability to make choices for the self despite possible peer group pressures reflects both the learning of positive social skills from possibly negative experiences and the development of maturity and independence in decision-making and behaviour. For instance, young people's views on sex and marriage showed an understanding that these relationships require a maturity of outlook, sound judgement, and time for relationships to mature. However, middle-class young people were more likely in general to perceive the values of deferring gratification within relationships, whereas working-class adolescents were generally more likely to report that they perceived sexual encounters as fairly inevitable and unromantic fumbling experiences that possibly led to early pregnancy and marriage. Nevertheless, it must be stated that an aspiration towards early marriage was not expressed by *any* of the mid-adolescent girls we talked with.

A number of issues seem relevant here. First, experimentation is an important process in gaining independence and responsibility for self-action. It is a step on the way to becoming more mature and adult-like and in learning to make choices and come to decisions. Second, as Coleman and Hendry (1990) have outlined, adults often give adolescents conflicting messages, different sets of expectations about both mature independence and childlike obedience in their behaviour. Hence young people struggle to gain independence and self-agency in a society riddled with many inconsistencies, few social 'signposts' to maturity, and major anomalies regarding rights and citizenship status (Jones and Wallace, 1992).

Thus, third, with regard to risk and risky health behaviours, adults can become very concerned – and over-anxious – on behalf of their adolescent offspring when 'catastrophes' occur. However, as Gore and Eckenrode (1994) stated, no issue is just one event! For example, a divorce can alter family relationships, change material circumstances, introduce 'strangers' into the family circle, create withdrawal and depression in one child, give another freedom from tensions and conflict and provide yet another with opportunities and challenges to become the new 'bread-winner'. Gore and Eckenrode suggest, therefore, that any event in a young person's life can be a challenge or a near immovable obstacle to further psycho-social development. The important elements of success or failure, according to Gore and Eckenrode are: the young person's competencies in perception, planning, decision-making, learning capacities and interpersonal skills that can be brought to bear on the issue, together with the prioritisation of key aspects of the tasks involved, and the appearance or absence of other concurrently stressful events. Their analysis of risk contexts and processes of skills and resilience development are useful extensions of Coleman's (1979) original focal theory of coping behaviours and 'overlap' of psycho-social difficulties in adolescence.

Lifestyles and health

The Young People's Leisure and Lifestyle Project (Hendry *et al.*, 1993b) showed various adolescent life trajectories which were fairly firmly embedded within social class boundaries. It was suggested, therefore, that in general terms, by mid-adolescence health behaviours and health concerns are essential component parts of a more holistic pattern of social class based lifestyles. In terms of Bronfenbrenner's ideas (1979) about individual development within socio-cultural settings, this would be where wider cultural norms filter down via community expectations and subcultural values to be translated into lifestyle developments by the individual's social behaviour and social learning in a variety of local contexts and social institutions. In turn, these lead to decision-making choices as various life events occur.

An alien race?

In a recent paper given at a conference on urban childhood Ulvik (1997) quotes the words of a Swedish folk singer, Olle Adolfson, from his song 'The Mysterious People':

Children are a people, and they live in a distant land.

In this depiction children are perceived as a strange tribe, hardly understandable to adults. It highlights a view that has gained currency, namely that it is pointless to assume simply that children are little adults. It has become accepted that children's perceptions, attitudes and patterns of reasoning are often distinct and very different. Sometimes the realisation of the very different ways in which young people construe and make sense of their lives has encouraged adults to identify children as a race apart, creatures from a parallel planet. There have been many good accounts in recent years of the ways in which we construct and reconstruct childhood (James and Prout, 1990). The cultural images which we use to describe children and childhood are important, as they give direction and shape to the attempts which we make to understand children's and young people's worlds. The changing cultural images of the child constitute what Wertsch (1991) has called 'cultural tools' shaping how children are seen by adults as well as by themselves.

It is clear that until very recently the way in which children were viewed by adults emphasised their powerlessness, their weakness, dependency and incompetence. Franklin (1995: 9) comments:

Definitions of a 'child' and 'childhood' entail more than a specification of an age of majority; they articulate society's values and attitudes towards children. They are typically disdaining and ageist.

The most popular recent discourses around childhood and youth would seem to move us towards a different conception of young people. Academics, policy makers and practitioners have all seemed keen to participate (in theory at least) in a new formulation which concerns the necessity to implement children's rights and to see each child as an individual, and there have been myriad calls for adults to start listening to 'children's voices', so that young people's perspectives can be used in planning interventions and programmes. The study from which this book results is just such a piece. Any such attempt must be applauded, because, as Lansdown comments:

> Children's views are still, for a substantial proportion of the adult population, often treated as ill-informed, irrational, irresponsible, amusing or cute. It is much more unusual for them to be given serious recognition, and then primarily when their views coincide with those of adults. (1996: 75)

We must not be fooled into thinking that this is a simple agenda, however. Simple vox-pop journalistic recordings of young voices are insufficient. There is not one *single* children's voice, a fact that we have attempted to demonstrate in this study. Young people's age, gender, social class, ethnicity and life experience all combine to give them as varied a set of 'voices' as would be expressed by the adult community.

Then, too, there is the fact that young people do not exist in childish worlds of their own, untouched by the constructions and discourses of the adult world with which they interact. As Bruner and Haste (1987) point out, meaning is constructed and negotiated in the way they live the child–adult interaction in their everyday lives. These interactions are discursive practices – ones where meaning is produced and constantly negotiated (Davies and Harre, 1990).

The third difficulty with which this new paradigm confronts us is that of how we respond to the identification of young people's perspectives. There have been warnings from many that it is insufficient for adults to listen to young people's voices and then to try to frame rights on their behalf (Waiton, 1995). Instead there is a call for responses which are empowering for young people themselves, leading them towards full participative citizenship. This raises immediate concerns for many observers. Just how competent are children and young people to take on these sorts of roles? Is this not just a way of abdicating our role as responsible adults or parents, and one that we will live to regret as we watch our young people possibly stumble and falter as they try to reinvent the wheel for themselves?

Descriptions of young people's transition to adulthood in the last few years have seen an increasing emphasis on the concept of citizenship as a desirable end goal of that maturational process (Jones and Wallace, 1992). Central to the notion of becoming a citizen is the idea that one's childhood and teenage years see a progressive gain in the development of various competencies, giving one also rights of self-determination and rightful access to a range of opportunity and institutional and welfare aid. In much of what has been written this transition is short-handed, using terms such as 'empowerment'.

Empowerment

We might pause here briefly to consider the concept of empowerment as it is currently construed in popular rhetoric and in the professional rhetoric of the caring services. We should also examine the way in which empowerment is now interpreted (in a new and non-reflexive sense) as a professional task of those working with young people in various welfare settings. So recent is this shift in popular perspective on the professional role of those working with young people that there has been little opportunity to evaluate the implications for the recipients of 'empowering practice'.

Research literature would seem to indicate that 'empowerment involves a more complicated set of processes than its invocation as a moral imperative implies' (Baistow, 1994: 35). Adams defines empowerment as 'the process by which individuals, groups and/or communities become able to take control of their circumstances and achieve their goals, thereby being able to work toward maximising the quality of their lives' (1990: 43). Such a definition captures the essential individualism of modern rhetoric. It is power over self rather than power over other individuals which is desirable. Control of self is emphasised and seen as good in itself.

A number of conflicting themes appear in the literature on empowerment. While the language used in identifying candidates for empowerment is often overtly political (Barr, 1995), for instance, the solutions suggested are often overwhelmingly psychological in tone (Stevenson and Parsloe, 1993). Moreover, the connections between individual empowerment and community or collective empowerment are implied but poorly explained.

Empowerment (rather like children's rights) is increasingly being seen as something done by professionals to people in need. Thus candidates for the empowerment activities of professionals might be the clients of health promoters, social workers, health visitors, youth workers and so on. They may also be consumers who should be able to exercise choice or rights. Such a formulation fits in with the agenda both of the new right with its free-market analysis as well as that of the liberal left with its needs-based consumerist analysis. Such articulations of the ideas around empowerment share common themes – solutions are seen as being ground level, bottom-up, localised, designed to increase user choice, participation and, critically, personal control.

We might ask how empowerment has come to have this new meaning, to have become something which is 'done unto' people by others in professional positions. Some have seen it as a reaction to the extent to which ordinary life has been colonised by professionals. Empowerment becomes a way of defining clients anew as consumers and of wresting some of the power away from professionals who were seen as having established an over-bureaucratic stranglehold on the organs of the welfare state. It is ironic, therefore, that 'far from being left roleless, or less powerful, by the process of empowerment, professionals are increasingly being seen as central to it in a number of ways which extend rather than reduce their involvement and interventions in the everyday life of citizens' (Baistow, 1994: 39).

These kinds of changes in the professional roles of workers in health and welfare agencies would seem to imply the need to acquire a whole different set of professional skills and know-how, and, on the part of the recipients, a new framework of relationships with workers. Despite much evidence in the professional literature urging the new paradigm, there is little material to date explaining how the desired outcomes might be achieved in practice or any indication of how these actions might make a difference in the lives of those candidates for empowerment.

This latter point has been explored a little by Beresford and Croft (1993), by Lord and McKillop Farlow (1990), and by Love and Hendry (1994), but they are almost alone in being concerned with the views of putative empowerment candidates. There is a dearth of research on user's experiences and views of empowerment. We simply do not know whether users desire empowerment or, if they do, whether their ideas about the nature of this are at odds with those of professionals. Our ignorance on this point is ironic in the context of the rhetoric about empowerment.

Given this ignorance there is a further danger that professional empowerment discourses will take the form of ones amenable to institutional organisation and evaluation, and that they will ignore the lessons from naturally occurring instances of mentoring and empowerment. Empirical studies tend to show that such instances occur in a voluntary setting, and are influenced by a level of empowerment beyond the individual psychology, that is, at a group or community level where experience has become collectivised and participative. Kieffer's (1984) model emphasises, for instance, that the empowerment process consists of several phases, the first of which he entitles 'entry'. Kieffer insists that the process of empowerment starts in a recognition by the individual of some challenge to his/her integrity – a threat to individual or familial self-interest. Kieffer maintains that the common daily experience of injustice or powerlessness is insufficient to trigger entry into the empowerment cycle. Similarly he feels that these initial reactions are never fostered by consciousness-raising, intellectual analysis or merely educative interventions. If this is true it poses interesting dilemmas for those working with young people within the new paradigm. Kieffer does, however, identify the central role of a mentor as a key link in the chain of a sustaining empowerment experience.

In a recent study Philip and Hendry (1997a) reflect on the fact that the most empowering examples of mentoring encountered by them in their research involved a much higher degree of reciprocity than is commonly found in worker–client relationships. Mentoring was seen to be a trigger for many young people to look for support elsewhere. Issues or problems once voiced to a supportive adult or same-near-age peer had become something that could be talked about, and young people were then happier to be referred on to another agency or individual for specialist advice or longer-term intervention. This project (Philip and Hendry, 1997b) provided evidence that mentoring gave young people some of the resilience or 'steeling mechanisms' that Rutter and Smith (1995) allude to in their work.

Concluding remarks

The study described in this book set out to explore young people's own feelings about their own health needs. Listening and responding to those voices will involve health workers themselves in developing different strategies towards the user groups of these services. Are those working with young people able to develop styles of operating which deliver true empowerment, or are notions of empowerment being slowly built into professional practice within an ironic new paradigm which does little to really connect with the health issues and problems young people have to surmount?

Such questions are critical in the lives of vulnerable young people. How can health educators and health promoters use these ideas to help young people through the transition points of their childhood and young adulthood?

We started this chapter by allowing one mid-adolescent to claim a degree of self-agency and the skills and abilities to behave sensibly in ways that are health-enhancing. We conclude this book by giving our support to the general principles behind the young person's 'message' to us. If health education is successfully to meet the needs of our young people, it is important that it is designed to encourage proactive behaviour in adolescents. Health educators can do this by providing non-judgemental knowledge, learning opportunities, and personal and social support networks. This would mean that young people make their own informed choices and decisions, and would be able to say, like our young interviewee: 'I won't do anything stupid.' And the reason why adolescents could say this would be because adult society has become sufficiently 'open' and collaborative with youth to enable them to have a future as genuine participants and to be considered, for the present, as learning partners with a voice in health concerns and social matters.

References

Aaro, L. E., Wold, B., Kannas, L. and Rimpela, M. (1986) 'Health behaviour in school-children. A WHO cross-national survey', *Health Promotion*, 1, 1: 17–33.

Abel, T. and McQueen, D. (1992) 'The formation of health lifestyles: a new empirical concept'. Paper presented to the BSA and ESMS Joint Conference on Health in Europe, Edinburgh, 18–21 September 1992.

Abrams, D., Abraham, C., Spears, R. and Marks, D. (1990) 'AIDS invulnerability: relationships, sexual behaviour and attitudes amongst 16–19 year olds', in P. Aggleton, P. Davies and G. Hart (eds) *AIDS: Individual, Cultural and Policy Dimensions*, London: Falmer Press.

Adams, G. R. (1983) 'Social competence during adolescence: social sensitivity, locus of control, empathy, and peer popularity', *Journal of Youth and Adolescence*, 12, 3: 203–211.

Adams, R. (1990) *Self-Help, Social Work and Empowerment*, London: Macmillan.

Aggleton, P., Toft, M. and Warwick, I. (1992) 'Working for young people: priorities for HIV/AIDS health promotion in local settings', in B. Evans, S. Sandberg and S. Watson (eds) *Working Where the Risks Are: Issues in HIV Prevention*, London: Health Education Authority.

Aldridge, J. and Becker, S. (1993) *Children Who Care: Inside the World of Young Carers*, Loughborough: Loughborough University Department of Social Sciences.

Almond, L. (1983) 'A guide to practice', *British Journal of Physical Education*, 14, 5: 134–135.

Altman, D. (1993) 'Expertise, legitimacy and the centrality of community', in P. Aggleton, P. Davies and G. Hart (eds) *AIDS: Facing the Second Decade*, London: Falmer.

Anderssen, N., Klepp, K.-I., Aars, H. and Jacobsen, R. (1994) 'Stability in physical activity levels in young adolescence: a two-year follow-up of the Norwegian Longitudinal Health Behaviour Study', *European Journal of Public Health*, 3: 175–180.

Backett, K. (1990) 'Image and reality. Health enhancing behaviours in middle class families', *Health Education Journal*, 49, 2: 61–63.

Backett, K. (1992a) 'The construction of health knowledge in middle class families', *Health Education Research*, 7: 497–507.

Backett, K. (1992b) 'Taboos and excesses: lay health moralities in middle class families', *Sociology of Health and Illness*, 14: 255–275.

Backett, K. and Alexander, H. (1991) 'Talking to young children about health: methods and findings', *Health Education Journal*, 50, 1: 34–38.

Backett, K. and Davison, C. (1992) 'Rational or reasonable? Perceptions of health at different stages of life', *Health Education Journal*, 51, 2: 55–59.

Baistow, K. (1994) 'Liberation and regulation? Some paradoxes of empowerment', *Critical Social Policy*, 42, 14: 34–46.

Bakken, L. and Romig, C. (1992) 'Interpersonal needs in middle adolescents: companionship, leadership and intimacy', *Journal of Adolescence*, 15, 3: 301–316.

Balding, J. (1986) 'Mayfly. A study of 1,237 pupils aged 14–15 who completed the Health Related Behaviour Questionnaire in May 1984'. Unpublished report. HEA Schools Health Education Unit, School of Education, University of Exeter.

Bancroft, J. (1990) 'The impact of socio-cultural influences on adolescent sexual development: further considerations', in J. Bancroft and M. Reinisch (eds) *Adolescence and Puberty*, Oxford: Oxford University Press.

Barnes, G. (1977) 'The development of adolescent drinking behaviour: an evaluative review of the impact of the socialisation process within the family', *Adolescence*, 12: 571–591.

Barr, M. (1995) 'Empowering communities: beyond fashionable rhetoric? Some reflections on the Scottish experience', *Community Development Journal*, 30, 2: 121–132.

Baumrind, D. (1967) 'Child care practices anteceding three patterns of pre-school behaviour', *Genetic Psychology Monographs*, 75: 43–88.

Baumrind, D. (1968) 'Authoritarian versus authoritative parent control', *Adolescence*, 3: 255–272.

Baumrind, D. (1971) 'Current patterns of parental authority', *Developmental Psychology Monograph*, 4: 1–102.

Beller, A. S. (1977) *Fat and Thin: A Natural History of Obesity*, New York: Farrar, Strauss and Giroux.

Beresford, P. and Croft, S. (1993) *Citizen Involvement – A Practical Guide for Change*, London: Macmillan.

Bibace, R. and Walsh, M. E. (1980) 'Development of children's concepts of illness', *Paediatrics*, 66: 912–917.

Biggs, S. J., Bender, M. and Foreman, J. (1983) 'Are there psychological differences between persistent solvent abusing delinquents and delinquents who do not use solvents?' *British Journal of Adolescence*, 6: 71–86.

Blaxter, M. (1987) 'Alcohol consumption', in B. D. Cox (ed) *The Health and Lifestyle Survey*, Cambridge: The Health Promotion Research Trust.

Blaxter, M. (1990) *Health and Lifestyles*, London: Routledge.

Blos, P. (1978) 'Children think about illness: their concepts and beliefs', in E. Gellert (ed.) *Psychosocial Aspects of Paediatric Care*, New York: Grune and Stratton.

Bø, I. (1995) 'The sociocultural environment as a source for growth among 15–16 year old boys', *Children's Environments*, 12, 4: 469–478.

Boskind-White, M. and White, W. C. (1987) *Bulimarexia: The Binge/Purge Cycle* (2nd edn), New York and London: Norton.

Bosma, H. A. (1992) 'Identity in adolescence: managing commitments', in G. R. Adams, T. Gullotta and R. Montemayor (eds) *Identity Formation During Adolescence*, Newbury Park: Sage.

Bourdieu, P. (1984) *Distinction: A Social Critique of the Judgement of Taste*, London: Routledge.

Brannen, J., Dodd, K., Oakley, A. and Storey, P. (1994) *Young People, Health and Family Life*, Milton Keynes: Open University Press.

Bridges Project (1988) *Fizz, Fat and Fasting*, Edinburgh: Bridges Project.

Bronfenbrenner, U. (1979) *The Ecology of Human Development*, Cambridge, Mass.: Harvard University Press.

Bruch, H. (1957) *The Importance of Overweight*, New York: W. W. Norton.

Bruch, H. (1985) 'Four decades of eating disorders', in D. M. Garner and P. E. Garfinkel (eds) *Handbook of Psychotherapy for Anorexia Nervosa and Bulimia*, New York: Guilford Press.

Bruchon-Schweitzer, M. (1990) *Une Psychologie du Corps*, Paris: PUF.

Bruner, J. and Hast, H. (1987) *Making Sense. The Child's Construction of the World*, London: Methuen.

Burt, C. E., Cohen, L. H. and Bjorck, J. P. (1988) 'Perceived family environment as a moderator of young adolescents' life stress adjustment', *American Journal of Community Psychology*, 16: 101–122.

Bury, J. (1984) *Teenage Pregnancy in Britain*, London: Birth Control Trust.

Bury, J. (1991) 'Teenager social behaviour and the impact of AIDS', *Health Education Journal*, 50, 1: 43–48.

Callaghan, G. (1992) 'Locality and localism', *Youth and Policy*, 39: 23–33.

Chisholm, L. and du Bois-Raymond, N. (1993) 'Youth transitions, gender and social change', *Sociology*, 27, 2: 259–279.

Coffield, F. (1992) 'Young people and illicit drugs', Summary Research Report. Northern Regional Health Authority and Durham University.

Coffield, F., Borrill, C. and Marshall, S. (1986) *Growing Up at the Margins*, Milton Keynes: Open University Press.

Coffield, F. and Gofton, L. (1994) *Drugs and Young People*, London: Institute for Public Policy Research.

Coggans, N. and McKellar, M. (1994) 'Drug use amongst peers: peer pressure or peer preference?' *Drugs: Education, Prevention and Policy*, 1, 1: 15–26.

Coggans, N., Shewan, D., Henderson, M. and Davies, J. B. (1991) 'Could do better – an evaluation of drug education', *Druglink*, Sept./ Oct.: 14–16.

Cohen, S. (1973) 'The volatile solvents', *Public Health Review*, 2, 2: 185–214.

Coleman, J. C. (ed.) (1979) *The School Years*, London: Methuen.

Coleman, J. C. and Coleman, E. Z. (1984) 'Adolescent attitudes to authority', *Journal of Adolescence*, 7: 131–141.

Coleman, J. C. and Hendry, L. B. (1990) *The Nature of Adolescence*, 2nd edn, London: Routledge.

Conger, J. T. and Petersen, A. C. (1984) *Adolescence and Youth*, New York: Harper and Row.

Cooter, R. (ed.) (1992) *In the Name of the Child: Health and Welfare 1880–1940*, London: Routledge.

CRDU (Children's Rights Development Unit) (1994) *The United Nations' Convention on the Rights of the Child: Briefing Papers*, London: CRDU.

Cresswell, T. (1992) 'Assessing community health and social needs in North Derbyshire using participatory rapid appraisal', *Community Health Action*, 24: 12–16.

Crisp, A. H. (1980) *Anorexia Nervosa: Let Me Be*, London: Plenum Press.

Crockett, L. J. and Petersen, A. C. (1987) 'Pubertal status and psychological development: findings from the early adolescence study', in R. M. Lerner and T. T. Foch (eds) *Biological and Psycho-Social Interactions in Early Adolescence: A Lifespan Perspective*, Hillsdale, NJ: Lawrence Erlbaum Associates.

Currie, C., McQueen, D. V. and Tyrrell, H. (1987) 'The First Year of the RUHBC/SHEG/WHO Survey of Health Behaviours of Scottish Schoolchildren', Edinburgh: Research Unit in Health and Behavioural Change.

Currie, C. and Todd, J. (1993) *Health Behaviours of Scottish School-children*. Report 3: *Sex Education, Personal Relationships, Sexual Behaviour and HIV/AIDS Knowledge and Attitudes*, Edinburgh: Research Unit in Health and Behavioural Change.

Currie, C., Todd, J. and Wijckmans, K. (1993) *Health Behaviours of Scottish Schoolchildren*. Report 2: *Family, Peer, School and Socio-economic Influences*, Edinburgh: Research Unit in Health and Behavioural Change.

Davies, J. and Coggans, N. (1991) *The Facts About Adolescent Drug Abuse*, London: Cassell.

Davies, M. and Harre, R. (1990) 'Positioning: the discursive production of selves', *Journal of the Theory of Social Behaviour*, 20, 1: 20–33.

Davis, J. (1990) *Youth and the Condition of Britain: Images of Adolescent Conflict*, London: Athlone Press.

Day, G. and Fitton, M. (1975) 'Religion and social status in rural Wales', *The Sociological Review*, 23, 4: 867–891.

Day, G. and Murdoch, J. (1993) 'Locality and community: coming to terms with place', *Sociological Review*, 41 (1): 82–111.

Devine, M. (1995) 'Health education: what do young people want to know?' *Interchange Series*, No. 31, Edinburgh: Scottish Office Education Department.

Diamond, A. and Goddard, E. (1995) *Smoking among Secondary School Children in 1994*, London: HMSO.

Di Clemente, R. J., Boyer, C. B. and Morales, E. S. (1988) 'Minorities and AIDS: knowledge, attitudes and misconceptions among Black and Latino adolescents', *American Journal of Public Health*, 78: 55–57.

Dielman, T. E., Leech, S., Becker, M. H., Rosenstock, I. M., Horvath, W. J. and Radius, S. M. (1992) 'Parental and child health beliefs and behaviour', *Health Education Quarterly*, 9, 2: 56–60.

Dishman, R. K. and Dunn, A. L. (1988) 'Exercise adherence in children and youth: implications for adulthood', in R. K. Dishmann (ed.) *Exercise Adherence. Its Impact on Public Health*, Champaign, IL: Human Kinetics Books.

Donaldson, M. (1978) *Children's Minds*, Glasgow: Fontana.

Dorn, N. (1983) *Alcohol, Youth and the State*, Oxford: Croom Helm.

Douglas, M. (1985) *Risk Acceptability According to the Social Sciences*, London: Routledge and Kegan Paul.

Duncan, P. D., Ritter, P. L., Dornbusch, S. M., Gross, R. T. and Carlsmith, J. M. (1985) 'The effects of pubertal timing on body-image, school behaviour and deviance', *Journal of Youth and Adolescence*, 14: 227–235.

Eagley, A. H., Ashmore, R. D., Makhijani, M. G. and Longo, L. C. (1991) 'What is beautiful is good, but . . .: A meta-analytic review of research on the physical attractiveness stereotype', *Psychological Bulletin*, 110: 109–128.

Eccles, J. S. and Midgley, C. (1989) 'Stage/environment fit: developmentally appropriate classrooms for early adolescents', in R. E. Ames and C. Ames (eds) *Research on Motivation in Education*, San Diego, CA: Academic Press.

Elkind, D. (1984) 'Teenage thinking: implications for health care', *Paediatric Nursing*, 10: 383–385.

Ericsson, K. A. and Simon, H. A. (1993) *Protocol Analysis: Verbal Reports as Data*, Cambridge, Mass.: MIT Press.

Erikson, E. (1968) *Identity: Youth in Crisis*, New York: Norton.

European Sports Charter (1975) *'Sport for All' Charter,* European Sports Ministers' Conference, Brussels.

Fallon, A. E. and Rozin, P. (1985) 'Sex differences in perceptions of desirable body shape', *Journal of Abnormal Psychology*, 31: 173–184.

Farquhar, C. (1990) *What Do Primary School Children Know about AIDS?* Working Paper No. 1, London: Thomas Coram Research Unit.

Farrell, C. (1978) *My Mother Said . . . The Way Young People Learned about Sex and Birth Control*, London: Routledge and Kegan Paul.

Fast Forward (1994a) *Headstrong? Peer Research Project Annual Report,* Edinburgh: Fast Forward Positive Lifestyles Ltd.

Fast Forward (1994b) *Sharing Works?* Edinburgh: Fast Forward Positive Lifestyles Limited.

Featherstone, M. (1991) 'The body in consumer culture', in M. Featherstone, M. Hepworth and B. S. Turner (eds) *The Body: Social Process and Cultural Theory*, London: Sage.

Fend, H. (1990) 'Ego-strength development and patterns of social relationships', in H. A. Bosma and A. E. Jackson (eds) *Coping and Self-concept in Adolescence*, Heidelberg: Springer-Verlag.

Ford, N. (1987) 'Research into heterosexual behaviour with

implications for the spread of AIDS', *British Journal of Family Planning*, 13: 50–54.

Ford, N. and Bowie, C. (1989) 'Urban-rural variations in the level of heterosexual activity of young people', *Area*, 21, 3: 237–248.

Ford, N. and Morgan, K. (1989) 'Heterosexual lifestyles of young people in an English city', *Journal of Population and Social Studies*, 1: 167–182.

Forth Valley Health Board (1993) *Health-related Behaviour of Young People in Schools in Central Region 1993*, Stirling: Directorate of Public Health Medicine, Forth Valley Health Board.

Franklin, B. (ed.) (1995) *The Handbook of Children's Rights*, London: Routledge.

Fraser, A., Gamble, L. and Kennett, P. (1991) 'Into the Pleasuredome', *Druglink*, 6, 6: 12–13.

Freire, P. (1972) *The Pedagogy of the Oppressed*, London: Penguin.

Frost, N. and Stein, M. (1989) *The Politics of Child Welfare*, Brighton: Harvester/Wheatsheaf.

Frost, N. and Stein, M. (1992) 'Empowerment and child welfare', in J. C. Coleman and C. Warren-Adamson (eds) *Youth Policy in the 1990s: The Way Forward*, London: Routledge.

Furlong, A., Biggart, A. and Cartmel, F. (1996) 'Neighbourhoods, opportunity structures and occupational aspirations', *Sociology*, 30, 3: 551–565.

Gans, H. (1962) 'Urbanism and suburbanism as ways of life', in A. Rose (ed.) *Human Behaviour and Social Processes*, London: Routledge and Kegan Paul.

Gardner, C. and Sheppard, J. (1989) *Consuming Passion, The Rise of Retail Culture*, London: Unwin Hyman.

Garner, C. L. (1989) *Does Deprivation Damage?* Report to the John Watson's Trust, University of Edinburgh Centre for Educational Sociology.

Garner, C. L. and Raudenbush, F. W. (1991) 'Neighbourhood effects on educational attainment: a multi-level analysis', *Sociology of Education*, 64: 251–262.

Gibbon, P. (1973) 'Arensberg and Kimball Revisited', *Economy and Society*, 4: 479–498.

Gilligan, C. (1990) 'Teaching Shakespeare's sister: notes from the underground of female adolescence', in C. Gilligan, N. P. Lyons and T. J. Hanover (eds) *Making Connections: The Relational World of Adolescent Girls at Emma Willard School*, Cambridge, Mass.: Harvard University Press.

Glendinning, A., Love, J., Shucksmith, J. and Hendry, L. B. (1992)

'Adolescence and health inequalities: extensions to McIntyre and West', *Social Science and Medicine*, 35, 5: 679–687.

Gochman, D. (1971) 'Some steps towards a psychological matrix for health behaviour', *Canadian Journal of Behavioural Science*, 3: 88–101.

Gochman, D. S. and Saucier, J. F. (1982) 'Perceived vulnerability in children and adolescents', *Health Education Quarterly*, 9, 2/3: 46–59.

Goddard, E. (1989) *Smoking among Secondary School Children in 1988*, OPCS Social Survey Division, London: HMSO.

Goddard, E. (1996) *Teenage Drinking in 1994*, London: HMSO.

Goffman, E. (1971) *The Presentation of Self in Everyday Life*, Harmondsworth: Pelican.

Gofton, L. (1990) 'On the town: drink and the "new lawlessness"', *Youth and Policy*, 29: 33–39.

Golding, J. (1987) 'Smoking', in B. D. Cox, *The Health and Lifestyle Survey*, Cambridge: The Health Promotion Research Trust.

Goldman, R. J. and Goldman, J. (1982) *Children's Sexual Thinking*, London: Routledge.

Gore, S. and Eckenrode, J. (1994) 'Context and process in research on risk and resilience', in R. J. Haggerty, L. R. Sherrod, N. Garmezy and M. Rutter (eds) *Stress, Risk, and Resilience in Children and Adolescents: Processes, Mechanisms, and Interventions*, New York: Cambridge University Press.

Grampian Health Board (1991) *Towards a Healthier Grampian Lifestyle*, Aberdeen: Departments of Public Health Medicine and Health Promotion, Grampian Health Board.

Grampian Health Board (1993) *Lifestyle Survey of Young People in Grampian,* Aberdeen: Grampian Health Board.

Greenfeld, D., Quinlan, D. M., Harding, P., Glass, E. and Bliss, A. (1987) 'Eating behaviour in an adolescent population', *International Journal of Eating Disorders*, 6: 99–111.

Griffin, C. (1993) *Representations of Youth*, London: Polity Press.

Griffin, C. (1988) 'Youth research, young women and the "gang of lads" model', in J. Hazerkarp, W. Meeus and Y. Te Poel (eds) *European Contributions to Youth Research*, Amsterdam: F.U. Press.

Griffiths, V. (1988) 'From "playing out" to "dossing out": young women and leisure', in E. Wimbush and M. Talbot (eds) *Relative Freedoms. Women and Leisure*, Milton Keynes: Open University Press.

Hedges, B. (1981) *Personal Leisure Histories*, London: Sports Council/ SSRC Panel.

Hein, K., Cohen, M. I. and Mark, A. (1978) 'Age at first intercourse among homeless adolescent females', *Journal of Paediatrics*, 93: 147–148.

Hendry, L. B., Glendinning, A., Shucksmith, J., Love, J. and Scott, J. (1993a) 'The developmental context of adolescent lifestyles', in R. Silbereisen and E. Todt (eds) *Adolescents in Context: The Interplay of Family, School, Peers and Work in Adjustment*, New York: Springer International.

Hendry, L.B. and Kloep, M. (1996) 'Is there life beyond "flow"?' Proceedings of 5th Biennial Conference of the EARA, University of Liège, May 1996.

Hendry, L. B., Shucksmith, J. and Love, J. G. (1989) *Young People's Leisure and Lifestyles*, Report of Phase 1 (1985–1989). Edinburgh: The Scottish Sports Council.

Hendry, L. B., Shucksmith, J., Love, J. G., and Glendinning, A. (1993b) *Young People's Leisure and Lifestyles*, London: Routledge.

Hendry, L. B., Shucksmith, J. and Philip, K. (1995) *Educating for Health: School and Community Approaches with Adolescents*, London: Cassell.

Hendry, L. B., Shucksmith, J., Philip, K. and Jones, L. (1991) 'Working with young people on drugs and HIV in Grampian Region'. Report of a research project for Grampian Health Board, University of Aberdeen: Department of Education:

Hepworth, M. and Featherstone, M. (1982) *Surviving Middle Age*, Oxford: Blackwell.

Hsu, L. K. G. and Holder, D. (1986) 'Bulimia nervosa: treatment and short term outcome', *Psychological Medicine*, 16: 6570.

Ives, R. (1990a) 'Sniffing out the solvent users', in M. Ashton (ed.) (1990) *Drug Misuse in Britain: National Audit of Drug Misuse Statistics*, London: Institute for the Study of Drug Dependence.

Ives, R. (1990b) 'The fad refuses to fade', *Druglink*, 5, 5: 12–13.

James, A. and Prout, A. (eds) (1990) *Constructing and Reconstructing Childhood: Contemporary Issues in the Sociological Study of Childhood*, London: Falmer Press.

Jenkins, R. (1983) *Lads, Citizens and Ordinary Kids: Working-class Youth Lifestyles in Belfast*, London: Routledge and Kegan Paul.

Johnson, A. M., Wadsworth, J., Wellings, K. and Field, J. (eds) (1994) *Sexual Attitudes and Lifestyles*, London: Blackwell.

Jones, G. and Wallace, C. (1992) *Youth, Family and Citizenship*, Milton Keynes: Open University Press.

Joseph, S. M. (1993) 'Childhood revisited: possibilities and predicaments in new research agendas', *British Journal of Sociology of Education*, 14, 1: 113–120.

Kalnins, I.V. and Love, R. (1982) 'Children's concepts of health and illness, and implications for health education: An overview', *Health Education Quarterly*, 9: 8–19.

Kalnins, I., McQueen, D. V., Backett, K. C., Curtice, L. and Currie, C. (1992) 'Children, empowerment and health promotion: some new directions in research and practice', *Health Promotion International*, 7, 1: 53–59.

Kandel, D. B. (1978) 'Homophilly selection and socialisation in adolescent friendships', *American Journal of Sociology*, 84: 427–436.

Kaufmann, F. X. (1990) *Zukunft der Familie*, München: Beck.

Kegeles, S. S. and Lund, A. K. (1982) 'Adolescents' health beliefs and acceptance of a novel preventive dental activity; replication and extension', *Health Education Quarterly*, 9, 2/3: 96–112.

Kelly, G. A. (1955) *The Psychology of Personal Constructs*, New York: Norton.

Kent-Baguley, P. (1990) 'Sexuality and youth work practice', in T. Jeffs and M. Smith (eds) *Young People, Inequality and Youth Work*, London: Macmillan.

Kieffer, C. H. (1984) 'Citizen empowerment: a developmental perspective on prevention in human services'. Special issue – *Studies in Empowerment: Steps Towards Understanding and Action*, 3, 2–3: 9–36.

Kirkwood, G. and Kirkwood, C. (1989) *Living Adult Education: Freire in Scotland*, Milton Keynes: Open University Press.

Kitwood, T. (1980) *Disclosures to a Stranger*, London: Routledge.

Klee, H. (1991) 'Sexual risk among amphetamine misusers: prospects for change'. Paper presented at the 5th Social Aspects of Aids Conference, London, March 1991.

Lacey, J. H. (1983) 'Bulimia nervosa, binge eating and psycho-genetic vomiting: a controlled treatment study and long-term outcome', *British Medical Journal*, 286: 1609–1613.

Lansdown, G. (1996) 'Respecting the rights of children to be heard', in G. Pugh (ed.) *Contemporary Issues in the Early Years*, London: Paul Chapman.

Lau, R. R., Quadrel, M. J. and Hartman, K. A. (1990) 'Development and change of young adults' preventive health beliefs and behaviour: influence from parents and peers', *Journal of Health and Social Behaviour*, 31, 3: 240–259.

Ledoux, S., Choquet, M. and Flament, M. (1991) 'Eating disorders among adolescents in an unselected French population', *International Journal of Eating Disorders*, 110: 81–89.

Lee, C. (1988) *Friday's Child: The Threat to Moral Education*, Wellingborough: Thorsons.

Lee, R. M. (1993) *Doing Research on Sensitive Topics*, London: Sage.

Lerner, R. M. (1985) 'Adolescent maturational changes and psychosocial development: a dynamic interactional perspective', *Journal of Youth and Adolescence*, 14: 355–372.

Lerner, R. M. and Karabenick, S. (1974) 'Physical attractiveness, body attitudes and self-concept in late adolescence', *Journal of Youth and Adolescence*, 14: 355–372.

Levin, L. L. (1989) 'Health for today's youth: hope for tomorrow's world', *World Health Forum*, 10, 2: 6–14.

Lewis, C. E. and Lewis, M. A. (1982) 'Children's health-related decision-making', *Health Education Quarterly*, 9, 2/3: 129–141.

Lord, C. and McKillop Farlow, M. (1990) 'A study of personal empowerment: implications for health promotion', *Health Promotion, Health and Welfare, Canada*, 29, 2: 1–8.

Love, J. and Hendry, L. B. (1994) 'Youth workers and young participants: two perspectives of youth work', *Youth and Policy* (Special issue, *New Directions in Youth Work*), 46: 43–55.

Maccoby, E. and Martin, J. (1983) 'Socialisation in the context of the family: parent–child interaction', in E. M. Hetherington (ed.) *Handbook of Child Psychology*, New York: Wiley.

McGurk, H. and Glachan, M. (1988) 'Children's conversation with adults', *Children and Society*, 2: 20–34.

MacIntyre, S. (1989) 'West of Scotland Twenty-07 Study: Health in the community', in C. Martin and D. McQueen (eds) *Readings for a New Public Health*, Edinburgh: Edinburgh University Press.

McKeganey, N. and Bloor, M. (1991) 'Spotting the invisible man: the influence of male gender on fieldwork relations', *British Journal of Sociology*, 42, 2: 195–210.

MacKintosh, A. M. and Eadie, D. R. (1993) 'Lifestyle and HIV/AIDS: A study of young people in Highland 1992–1993', Glasgow: Centre for Social Marketing, University of Strathclyde.

Magnusson, D., Stattin, H. and Allen, V. L. (1985) 'Biological maturation and social development. A longitudinal study of some adjustment processes from mid-adolescence to adulthood', *Journal of Youth and Adolescence,* 14: 267–283.

Marcia, J. E. (1980) 'Identity in adolescence', in J. Adelson (ed.) *Handbook of Adolescent Psychology*, New York: Wiley.

Marsh, A., Dobbs, J. and White, A. (1986) *Adolescent Drinking*, OPCS Social Survey Division, London: HMSO.

Masterson, G. (1979) 'The management of solvent abuse', *British Journal of Adolescence*, 2: 65–75.

Mayall, B. (1994) *Negotiating Health: Primary School Children at Home and School*, London: Cassell.

Mead, G. H. (1934) *Mind, Self and Society*, Chicago, IL: University of Chicago Press.

Meeus, W. (1989) 'Parental and peer support in adolescence', in K. Hurrelman and U. Engel (eds) *The Social World of Adolescents*, Berlin: de Gruyter.

Melton, G. B., Levine, R. J., Koocher, G. P., Rosenthal, R. and Thompson, W. C. (1988) 'Community consultation in socially sensitive research: lessons from clinical trials for treatment for AIDS', *American Psychologist*, 43: 573–581.

Michell, L. and West, P. (1997) 'Peer pressure to smoke: the meaning depends on the method', *Health Education Research: Theory and Practice*, 11, 1: 14–25.

Moore, S. and Rosenthal, D. (1993) *Sexuality in Adolescence*, London: Cassell.

MORI (1989) *Ten Years On*, London: MORI.

MORI (1990) *Young Adult's Health and Lifestyles*. Research conducted for Health Education Authority, London: MORI.

Murray, S. A., Tapson, J., Turnbull, L., McCallum, J. and Little, A. (1994) 'Listening to local voices: adapting rapid appraisal to assess health and social needs in general practice', *British Medical Journal*, 308: 698–700.

Natapoff, J. N. (1982) 'A developmental analysis of children's ideas of health', *Health Education Quarterly*, 9, 2/3: 34–35.

Newman, B. A. and Murray, C. (1983) 'Identity and family relations in early adolescence', *Journal of Early Adolescence*, 3: 293–303.

Nichols, A. K. and Mahoney, C. A. (1989) 'Fitness and activity evaluation in school children', in Health Promotion Research Trust, *Fit for Life: Proceedings of a Symposium on Fitness and Leisure*, Cambridge: Health Promotion Research Trust.

Nisbet, J. and Shucksmith, J. (1986) *Learning Strategies*, London: Routledge and Kegan Paul.

Noller, P. and Callan, V. (1991) *The Adolescent in the Family*, London: Routledge.

Nottelmann, E. D., Susman, E. J., Inoff-Germain, G., Cutler, G. B. Jnr, Loriaux, D. L. and Chrousos, G. P. (1987) 'Developmental processes in early adolescence: relations between adolescent adjustment problems and chronologic age, pubertal stage, and puberty-related serum hormone levels', *Journal of Pediatrics*, 110: 473–480.

O'Bryan, L. (1989) 'Young people and drugs', in S. MacGregor (ed.) *Drugs and British Society: Responses to a Social Problem in the Eighties*, London: Routledge.

Oosterwegel, A. and Oppenheimer, L. (1990) 'Concepts within the self-concept: a developmental study on differentiation', in L. Oppenheimer (ed.) *The Self-concept: European Perspective on its Development, Aspects and Applications*, Heidelberg: Springer-Verlag.

Orkney Health Board (1993) *Lifestyle Survey of Young People in Orkney*, Executive Summary, Kirkwall: Health Promotion Department, Orkney Health Board.

Pahl, R. (1966) 'The rural urban continuum', *Sociologia Ruralis*, 6, 3/4: 142–163.

Palmer, R., Oppenheimer, R., Dignon, A., Chalones, D. and Howells, K. (1990) 'Childhood sexual experience with adults, reported by women with eating disorders', *The British Journal of Psychiatry*, 156: 699–703.

Palmonari, A., Pombeni, M. L. and Kirchler, E. (1989) 'Peer groups and the evolution of self-esteem in adolescence', *European Journal of Psychology of Education*, 4: 3–15.

Petosa, R. (1989) 'Adolescent wellness: implications for effective health education programmes', *Health Values*, 13, 5: 492–494.

Philip, K. and Hendry, L. B. (1997a) 'Young people and mentoring: towards a typology', *Journal of Adolescence*, 19: 43–62.

Philip, K. and Hendry, L. B. (1997b) *Young People, Mentoring and Youth Work*, Report to the Johann Jakobs Foundation, Zurich.

Plant, M. and Plant, M. (1992) *Risk-Takers. Alcohol, Drugs, Sex and Youth*, London: Routledge.

Qvortrup, J. (1990) 'A voice for children in statistical and social accounting: a plea for children's rights to be heard', in A. James and A. Prout (eds) *Constructing and Reconstructing Childhood: Contemporary Issues in the Sociological Study of Childhood*, Basingstoke: Falmer Press.

Qvortrup, J. (1995) 'Childhood and modern society: a paradoxical relationship?' in J. Brannen and M. O'Brien (eds) *Childhood and Parenthood. Proceedings of ISA Committee for Family Research Conference on Children and Families, 1994*, Institute of Education, University of London.

Ramsey, B. (1990) 'Dangerous games: UK solvent deaths 1983–1988', *Druglink*, 5, 5: 8–9.

Reay, D. (1996) 'Contextualising choice: social power and parental involvement', *British Educational Research Journal*, 22, 5: 581–598.

Redhead, S. (1993) *Rave Off: Politicised Deviance in Contemporary Youth Culture*, Aldershot: Avebury.

Ribbens, J. (1995) 'Mothers' images of children and their implications for maternal responses', in J. Brannen and M. O'Brien (eds) *Childhood and Parenthood. Proceedings of ISA Committee for Family Research Conference on Children and Families, 1994.* Institute of Education, University of London.

Roberts, K. (1968) 'The entry into employment: an approach towards a general theory', *Sociological Review* 16: 165–184.

Roberts, K. (1975) 'The developmental theory of occupational choice: a critique and an alternative', in G. Esland, G. Salaman and M. Speakman (eds) *People and Work*, Edinburgh: Holmes McDougall.

Rodriguez-Tomé, H. (1972) *Le moi et l'autre dans la conscience de l'adolescent*, Neuchâtel: Delachaux et Niestlé.

Rodriguez-Tomé, H. and Bariaud, F. (1984) 'Self-identity and self-knowledge in adolescence'. Paper presented at First European Conference on Developmental Psychology, Groningen.

Rodriguez-Tomé, H. and Bariaud, F. (1990) 'Anxiety in adolescence: sources and reactions', in H. A. Bosma and A. E. Jackson (eds) *Coping and Self-Concept in Adolescence*, Heidelberg: Springer-Verlag.

Rosen, G. and Ross, A. (1968) 'Relationship of body image to self concept', *Journal of Consulting and Clinical Psychology*, 32: 100.

Rosenstock, I. M., Strecher, V. J. and Becker, M. H. (1988) 'Social learning theory and the health belief model', *Health Education Quarterly*, 15, 2: 175–183.

Rotherham-Borus, M. J., Becker, J. V., Koopman, C. and Kaplan, M. (1991) 'AIDS knowledge and beliefs, and sexual behaviour of sexually delinquent and non-delinquent (runaway) adolescents', *Journal of Adolescence*, 14: 199–244.

RUHBC (1993a) *Health Behaviours of Scottish Schoolchildren: Report 2 – Family, Peer, School and Socio-economic Influences*. Edinburgh: Research Unit in Health and Behavioural Change.

RUHBC (1993b) *Health Behaviours of Scottish Schoolchildren: Report 3 – Sex Education, Personal Relationships, Sexual Behaviour and HIV/ AIDS Knowledge and Attitudes*. Edinburgh: Research Unit in Health and Behavioural Change.

Rutter, M. and Smith, D. (1995) *Psychosocial Disorders in Young People: Time Trends and Their Causes*, London: Wiley.

Schofield, M. (1965) *The Sexual Behaviour of Young People*, London: Longman.

Scott, J., Brynin, M. and Smith, R. (1994) *The British Household Panel Study (Youth Survey)*. Interim report for the HEA Family Health Research Programme, ESRC Research Centre on Micro-Social Change in Britain: University of Essex.

Secretary of State for Health (1991) *The Health of the Nation* (Cm 1523), London: HMSO.

Sgritta, G. B. and Saporiti, A. (1989) 'Myth and reality in the discovery and representation of childhood', in P. Close (ed.) *Family Divisions and Inequalities in Modern Society*, London: Macmillan.

Sharp, D. and Lowe, G. (1989) 'Adolescents and alcohol – a review of the recent British research', *Journal of Adolescence*, 12: 295–307.

Shaw, M. (1984) *Sport and Leisure Participation and Lifestyles in Different Residential Neighbourhoods. An Exploration of the ACORN Classification*, London: Sports Council.

Shucksmith, J. (1994) *Young People, Families and Alcohol: A Literature Review*, Edinburgh: Health Education Board for Scotland.

Shucksmith, J. and Philip, K. (1994) 'Between the devil and the deep blue sea: teachers' responses to teaching HIV'. Paper given at British Sociological Association conference, Manchester, UK.

Shucksmith, J., Hendry, L. B. and Glendinning, A. (1995) 'Models of parenting: implications for adolescent well-being within different types of family contexts', *Journal of Adolescence*, 18: 253–270.

Silbereisen, R. K. and Noack, P. (1990) 'Adolescents' orientations for development', in H. A. Bosma and A. E. Jackson (eds) *Coping and Self-Concept in Adolescence*, Heidelberg: Springer-Verlag.

Silverman, D. (1993) *Interpreting Qualitative Data: Methods for Analysing Talk, Text and Interaction*, London: Sage.

Simmons, R. and Rosenberg, S. (1975) 'Sex, sex roles and self image', *Journal of Youth and Adolescence*, 4: 229–256.

Simmons, R. G. and Blyth, D. A. (1987) *Moving into Adolescence: The Impact of Pubertal Change and School Context*, New York: Aldine de Gruyter.

Simmons, R. G., Blyth, D. A. and McKinney, K. L. (1983) 'The social and psychological effects of puberty on white females', in J. Brooks-Gunn and A. Petersen (eds) *Girls at Puberty: Biological and Psychosocial Perspectives*, New York: Plenum.

Stacey, B. and Davies, J. (1970) 'Drinking behaviour in childhood and adolescence: an evaluative review', *British Journal of Addiction*, 65: 203–212.

Stattin, H. and Magnusson, D. (1990) *Pubertal Maturation in Female Development*, Hillsdale, NJ: Lawrence Erlbaum Associates.

Stegen, W. (1983) 'Sexual experience and contraceptive practice of young women attending a youth advisory clinic', *British Journal of Family Planning*, 8: 138–139.

Steinberg, L. D. and Silverberg, S. B. (1986). 'The vicissitudes of autonomy in early adolescence', *Child Development*, 57: 841–851.

Stevenson, O. and Parsloe, P. (1993) *Community Care and Empowerment*, York: Joseph Rowntree Foundation.

Streitmatter, J .L. (1985) 'Cross-sectional investigation of adolescent perceptions of gender roles', *Journal of Adolescence*, 8: 183–193.

Tajfel, H. (ed.) (1982) *Social Identity and Intergroup Relations*, Cambridge: Cambridge University Press.

Tiggemann, M. and Pennington, B. (1990) 'The development of gender differences in body-size dissatisfaction', *Australian Psychologist*, 25: 306–313.

Tobin, J. W. (1985) 'How promiscuous are our teenagers? A survey of teenage girls attending a family planning clinic', *British Journal of Family Planning*, 10: 107–112.

Ulvik, O. S. (1997) 'Discourses of childhood – perspectives of children committed to care by the child welfare'. Paper given at Urban Childhood Conference, Trondheim, Norway, June 1997.

Waiton, S. (1995) 'When children's rights are wrong', *Scottish Child*, December 1994/January 1995: 14–16.

Wallace, C. and Cross, M. (1990) *Youth in Transition: The Sociology of Youth and Youth Policy*, Basingstoke: Falmer.

Warwick, I., Aggleton, P. and Homans, H. (1988) 'Constructing commonsense – young people's beliefs about AIDS', *Sociology of Health and Illness*, 10, 3: 213–233.

Wellings, K. and Bradshaw, S. (1994) 'First heterosexual intercourse', in A. M. Johnson, J. Wadsworth, K. Wellings and J. Field (eds), *Sexual Attitudes and Lifestyles*, London: Blackwell.

Wertsch, J. (1991) *Voices of the Mind. A Sociocultural Approach to Mediated Action*, London: Harvester/Wheatsheaf.

Whichelow, M. J. (1987) 'Dietary habits', in B. D. Cox (ed.) *The Health and Lifestyle Survey*, Cambridge: Health Promotion Research Trust.

Wight, D. (1990) 'The impact of HIV/AIDS on young people's sexual behaviour in Britain: a literature review', Working Paper No. 20, Glasgow: Medical Research Council, Medical Sociology Unit.

Wight, D. (1993) 'Constraints or cognition? Young men and safer heterosexual sex', in P. Aggleton, P. Davies and G. Hart (eds) *AIDS: The Second Decade*, Basingstoke: Falmer Press.

Williams, J., Wetton, N. and Moon, A. (1989) *A Picture of Health. What Do You Do That Makes You Healthy and Keeps You Healthy?* London: Health Education Authority.

Wright, S. P. (1991) *Trends in Deaths Associated with Abuse of Volatile Substances 1971–1989*, London: St George's Hospital Medical School.

Young Scot (1993) Issue No. 17, Edinburgh: Scottish Community Education Council.

Youniss, J. and Smollar, J. (1985) *Adolescent Relations with Mothers, Fathers and Friends*, Chicago, IL: University of Chicago Press.

Youniss, J. and Smollar, J. (1990) 'Self through relationship development', in H. A. Bosma and A. E. Jackson (eds) *Coping and Self-concept in Adolescence*, Heidelberg: Springer-Verlag.

Zinneker J. (1990) 'Vom Strassenkind zum verhauslichten Kind. Kindheitsgeschichte im Prozess der Zivilisation', in I. Behnke (Hsrg.), *Stadtgesellschaft und Kindheit im Prozess der Zivilisation*, Opladen: Leske and Budrich.

Subject index

Name index